IDEAL, FACT, AND MEDICINE

A Philosophy for Health Care

Charles J. Dougherty

UNIVERSITY
PRESS OF
AMERICA

LANHAM • NEW YORK • LONDON

174.2
D74
Q

Library of Congress Cataloging in Publication Data

Dougherty, Charles J., 1949-
  Ideal, fact, and medicine.

  Bibliography: p.
  1. Medical ethics. 2. Medicine—Philosophy.
I. Title.
R724.D68   1985   174'.2   85-6124
ISBN 0-8191-4657-9 (alk. paper)
ISBN 0-8191-4658-7 (pbk. : alk. paper)

All University Press of America books are produced on acid-free
paper which exceeds the minimum standards set by the National
Historical Publications and Records Commission.

for
Constance Marie
and
Justin Charles

TABLE OF CONTENTS

INTRODUCTION

This is a book in medical ethics, a book that has grown out of my experience as a philosopher teaching in the field. It is written for persons working in the health care professions, those studying for these professions, and the rest of us who are served by these professionals. It is a hard book because the issues at hand are hard. But it is also a simple book; one that is jargon free and straightforward and that tries to be both coherent and enlightening.

The book addresses contemporary health care professionals as I have come to see them: persons with profound moral commitments but deep skepticism about moral discourse, with extraordinary intelligence but underdeveloped reasoning skills, with great respect for technology but a keen fear of its abuse, with an exceptional sense of fact but a confused sense of vision. Above all, contemporary health care professionals appear to know that what they do is of immeasurable human importance but doubt they can articulate that importance and fear they cannot direct its future. If this work can be of help to them it will have justified itself.

This book also tries to complement a growing philosophical literature in medical ethics and the philosophy of medicine. Much of that literature is composed of article length analyses of controversies in medicine. These analyses are often gathered together in collections which present an evenhanded look at the several ethical perspectives which may be urged on a given controversy. This approach has been good for medicine since it has provided an important reflective element in the biomedical debates of the last decade and will surely contribute similarly into the future. This approach has also been good for philosophy since it has provided an opportunity for philosophers to engage particular problems of life in a relatively well defined practical context. Against this background, I have written a book which is, instead, synthetic; a book which constructs a larger framework for understanding and appreciating, not so much the controversies of medicine, but the personal and social nature of what medical care is or could be. To do this, I have found it necessary to begin with accounts of philosophy itself, of what we are as persons in society, and of morality and ethics.

This book is also meant to be of value to the lay person. We have all become dependent on health care professionals and health care institutions. Our births, deaths, and many of the most important events in between are tied to these professionals and institutions. It is part of the argument of this book that health care professionals and their institutions are meant to serve individual persons in the public at large, and that this service should be based on a profound respect for the rights of patients. If this book can contribute to a better understanding among patients and potential patients of their relationship with health care professionals and institutions and the rights they may justly demand, it will have served one of its main purposes.

i

The book has four parts. In the first part, the nature of philosophical reflection is discussed and it is shown how such reflection can be relevant to the affairs of the world. Next, a general characterization of reality as composed of both our human ideals and the world of fact is offered. Against that background, some key features of our nature as human beings are explored, and two ideals which dominate the rest of the book are evolved: the ideals of autonomous persons in progressive societies.

In part two, morality and ethics are considered as tools for the realization of these ideals in fact. Morality is described as an intuitive and emotive system of habitual judgments of value and duty. Ethics is then defined as a rational reflection on concrete moral experience. Finally, a normative ethical framework is put forth; an ethic of maximizing, in order, persons' practical autonomy, happiness, and pleasure within the prior constraint of respect for human rights.

Part three begins the use of the tools of morality and ethics on behalf of the ideals of autonomous persons in progressive societies. Sickness and wellness are described and some consequences of these descriptions are drawn. The character of the relationship between health care professional and patient is then outlined and some recommendations on medical education are offered. These insights are then applied to the medical care of children and adults with diminished autonomy.

In part four, certain social dimensions of medicine are considered. The character of the hospital experience is described with special attention to the legal rights of hospital patients. Next, the ethical issues raised by the use of human persons as research subjects are examined. This social perspective ends with a look at some of the promises and perils of our growing genetic knowledge and power.

It is also part of the argument of the book that human persons are inherently social. The achievement of any one of us is also the achievement of the other persons and societies from which that one has come. So it is with this book. What wisdom there may be in the following pages is largely the wisdom of others. I am conscious of great intellectual debts to Charles Sanders Peirce, John Dewey, Immanuel Kant, Aristotle, and to the many others I have named where appropriate. I owe a rather large and specific intellectual debt to my wife, Sandra L. Dougherty, J.D., who did most of the research on hospital patients' legal rights and who collaborated with me in an earlier effort in this area. I know I have many other intellectual debts I am unconscious of, thoughts I owe to others, but thoughts I have lived with so long as to think my own.

I am grateful for the support of my family and friends, my former teachers, and my colleagues at Creighton University. I thank the Graduate School at Creighton University for the financial and technical support that made writing this book possible, and the people who helped me prepare its final form, especially Darlis Vauble and Peggy Troy. I am particularly grateful to the many health sciences students I have taught and who have taught me; students who were gracious enough to share their clinical experiences with me and unabashed enough to tell me when I was factually wrong about some medical technology or some dimension of a clinical relationship. This is a better book for their efforts.

I. The Ideal: Personal Autonomy In Progressive Societies

Chapter 1

The Function and Limits of Speculation

A. The Nature of Philosophy

This is a speculative book about the nature of the human person and human societies and about our experiences of morality and ethics. This is also a practical book about the relevance of these speculations for understanding and improving the character of contemporary medical care. It is a philosophical book about ideals and facts: the ideals of autonomous persons in progressive societies and the facts of what facilitates or frustrates these ideals in medical contexts. The hope that animates this whole inquiry is that philosophical speculation on our ideals can help us to clarify, organize, and criticize the world of facts in such a way as to bring about a greater realization of those ideals in fact. Since the possibility of this practical result depends on the success of the prior speculation, it will be useful to begin with an account of what philosophy is, and how it allows for the speculations and applications which follow.

The question, what is philosophy?, is a curious one at the outset since it is itself a philosophical question. The question, what is chemistry?, by contrast, is not itself a chemical question but one that is preparatory and external to the business of chemistry. One does no work in chemistry by merely learning what chemistry is. The same or similar points can be made about other disciplines. What is psychology?, is not itself a psychological issue. What is history?, what is biology?, what is the law, medicine, business management? — all of these are questions preparatory and external to the study of the discipline at hand and not questions internal to their disciplines. This is not the case with philosophy. By its very nature, philosophy breaks down the distinction between external and preparatory issues and questions proper to the discipline itself. To describe the nature of philosophy is already to reflect philosophically.

Because this is so, because there is no intellectually external ground on which to stand before philosophy begins, to describe the nature of philosophy is to take a position within philosophy itself. Now there can be no denying the lack of consensus among philosophers on philosophical questions, even on the most elementary questions. To compare philosophy to other disciplines again, one expects most chemists to agree on the fundamentals of chemistry, most psychologists to agree on the essentials of psychology, most historians to agree on the rudiments of history, etc. There is no similar agreement among philosophers. Therefore, to describe the nature of philosophy is to reflect philosophically and to reflect philosophically is to assert views not necessarily held by all competent philosophers. Thus the reader is provided fair warning at the start. While what follows is not wildly idiosyncratic nor unrelated to the views of many other philosophers and many great philosophical traditions, what follows is the philosophical position of one philosopher on the nature of philosophy.[1] How and why this can be so should be clearer shortly.

Philosophy, on this account, is the use of wonder for the sake of attaining wisdom. It is the profoundly personal asking of intelligent why's in the pursuit of wisdom for oneself and one's society.

Philosophy deals with profound issues, issues which shape human lives and give them coherence and direction. Philosophy wonders at these issues and uses that wonder to investigate what truly matters in life from the things that make our lives worth living to the things that make our deaths meaningful. Because philosophy wonders at what truly matters, the issues it raises are deep both cognitively and emotively. There is no need to catalogue philosophical issues to make this point as it is clear already by the themes at hand here: who are we as human persons?, what is the nature and significance of our moral experience?, how should beings such as ourselves with the moral experience we have relate to one another in contexts of medical care? These are not easy nor surface questions. As philosophical questions, they are profound; they have the qualities of seriousness and depth; they are both thought and felt keenly.

These questions are also personal. They relate directly to the individual person who asks them earnestly. Philosophical questions are questions about **my** life and about **yours.** Since philosophy is directed toward the lives of persons, it can be no more objective than the character of our personal lives, lives marked and made significant by the internal, by the subjective. Philosophy is a personal discipline and not an impartial science. It calls for personal judgments one can only make for oneself. Thus, it will not be enough for the reader to merely read along, memorize key points, or observe my thought objectively. If this work is to be successful as a philosophical reflection, it must be challenged and engaged at the subjective level of one's personal existence. If this is to be a philosophical reflection for you, the reader, you must make it your own.

The lack of consensus among philosophers on key philosophical questions provides a point of departure for the next element of philosophy: the wondering of philosophy expresses itself in an activity of question asking. Philosophers with differing substantive views in philosophy can recognize one another as philosophers nonetheless because arriving at substantive answers in philosophy is not nearly as important as is the asking of philosophical questions. As an expression of a stance of wondering, asking questions in this context does not simply mean articulating interrogatives. The asking of philosophical questions engages a process of intellectual exploration, a quest for greater understanding, appreciation, and insight. This asking may proceed with a wondering and questioning stance even when interrogatives are not used explicitly. Even when philosophers construct systematic answers, these answers can be regarded as extended questions themselves. "Perhaps," "it seems so," "it appears that," "maybe" — these words and their like display the wondering attitude of philosophy even in the midst of the construction of answers to the questions asked. Philosophers do offer answers to their questions, of course. But this product of philosophy, as precious as it can be, is not nearly so valuable as the process of asking questions itself. Answers to the central questions of human existence can shape and have shaped the character of individual human lives and whole civilizations, but they come and go; they change as the ideals and the facts of persons and civilizations change. By contrast, the activity of asking philosophical questions is insistent, perennial, and far more definitively a mark of the human species than any proposed set of answers. This is so because the asking of philosophical questions expresses a peculiarly human sense of wonder at the world around us and within us. Philosophy wonders not only at life's obvious mysteries, at the facts of our births, our deaths, at the marvels of the natural world. Philosophy also wonders at the mysteries inherent in the ordinary, at the fact of being a person, at the human senses of value and duty, at the marvels of communication and action in our social world. Thus philosophy enriches the character of experience with a pervasive sense of wonder by its very activity of question asking and by the construction of answers which broaden and deepen the questions themselves.

Yet the activity of philosophy is no random generation of questions. Though it shares in the wonderment of childhood, it is not childlike in method. Philosophy seeks to be intelligent. Its explorations are orderly, coherent, and systematic in intention. This does not entail that philosophy rejects the life of the emotions or employs the method of a computer. The intelligence of philosophy is open to all phenomena, cognitive and emotive, and its logic is the thoroughly human one of observing, guessing, drawing reasonable implications, and checking these implications with experience. Most of all, the intelligence of philosophy lies in its direct appeal to the common experience of human beings. Philosophical reflection is a profound and personal activity but it binds itself by standards wider than the exclusively subjective. It seeks a truth both subjectively significant for the individual person and intersubjectively available to other persons as well. Because of this, philosophy embodies the intelligence of human conversation itself: sometimes distorted, sometimes a bit too private, but always in search of meaningful and clear communication.

The very core of philosophy is the why question. This means not only the question which literally begins with the word 'why.' It also means the inquiry with a why structure, the investigation which examines our most

3

fundamental assumptions in a radical fashion. A why inquiry avoids the peripheral and goes straight to the very heart of matters. It examines the bases of our most central assumptions, those on which so many other judgments routinely depend. Imagine someone asserting, for example, that all persons must be autonomous, or must fulfill their promises, or must care for other human persons. Now imagine a second person simply asking "why?" to these assertions. This why question is a challenge to the world of the assertions made, an implicit critique, a demand for reasons and justification. Such a mode of examination has radical implications. Since most of the fundamental questions of life are presented to us as solved, that is, as nonquestions by our parents, by our religions, and by our cultures generally; philosophy is a potentially subversive discipline. It calls on us to question what is most uncomfortable for us to question, viz. the most fundamental assumptions of our personal and social lives. It suggests that things might be another way or no way at all. Thus, philosophy goes to the roots of things. It is the most radical of disciplines.

But this radical questioning, though potentially subversive in itself, is not engaged in for the sake of intellectual destruction. It is easy to attack a set of beliefs and assumptions with a series of unrelenting whys. The more difficult philosophical task is to use such questions, the answers they suggest, and the further questions these answers in turn provoke as a way of pursuing wisdom. Philosophers, by definition, are lovers of wisdom, not lovers of the subversion of assumptions. Philosophy uses wonder to examine assumptions in the most radical way possible as a means of seeking wisdom. Since philosophers use their methods to pursue, to seek, to love wisdom, they admit by implication that they do not have and possess the full wisdom they desire. Exactly what constitutes wisdom is perhaps the most difficult philosophical issue of all and those who seek it while not having it must be reluctant to characterize it fully. Still, some tentative things can be said of it. Wisdom is not to be found only in an other worldly knowledge of truth in the ideal, nor in immersion into the wholly factual doings of the world. Instead, wisdom integrates ideal and fact. It is the skill of interpreting the factual events of daily life in terms of an intelligent ideal worldview and of using this interpretation as the basis for making good decisions. This is the goal of philosophy and it cannot be arrived at by the merely subversive use of why questions. Radical questioning is thus not an end in itself but a means of expressing a wonder which, it is hoped, will help to secure a greater portion of wisdom. And wisdom can be increased only if one is prepared to offer some answers, however tentative and questioning in themselves, to the radical questions raised. Wonder gives way to wisdom as why's give way to maybe's.

Finally, philosophy is both personal and social. The wisdom philosophy seeks is a most general and therefore most useful skill which can be applied to an individual's life and the life of society as well. Perhaps one of the first bits of wisdom one can learn through philosophy is that the distinction between self and society, while real, is not as exclusive a distinction as it may appear. A wise person is the achievement of many societies, of a

4

family, a neighborhood, a nation, a culture. A wise society is both the expression of multiple acts of personal wisdom and the horizon against which more wise persons are made in the future. A knowledge of truth in the ideal, a sense of fact in the concrete, and the skill to integrate the two into sound decision-making are marks of human excellence whether they are achieved in an individual's life or in that of a whole society. Philosophy seeks such excellence for person and society.

Given this understanding of philosophy, it is easy to see why philosophy is at once thoroughly abstract and yet thoroughly relevant. Philosophy explores the abstract and ideal for the sake of its ultimate practical relevance to the living of a human life in all of its multiple factual dimensions. Thus philosophy is equally at home in an armchair and in the marketplace, in speculation and in application. Its most fundamental tenet is that reflection born in wonder can make an active difference for the better in our lives. Philosophy therefore is a liberal art; it can liberate persons and societies from the tyranny of unexamined assumptions and the bad decisions which follow from them. Philosophy is also one of the humanities; it can offer a richer appreciation of ourselves and our world by provoking a generalized sense of wonder at all things human and related to the human. And as the radical pursuit of wisdom that it is, philosophical reflection can afford us an opportunity to better understand ourselves as persons in societies and to act in light of that better understanding. It is the hope of this endeavor that such an abstract, philosophical understanding can help us make wiser decisions in the concrete personal and social interactions of the contemporary medical context.

B. Whole and Part; Real and Ideal

Having seen something of the character of philosophical reflection in general, we can turn now to a consideration a bit more specific. How is it possible to reflect in such a manner and how are we enabled to improve the character of our practical decision-making by so doing?

Let us begin with this assertion: Life as it is lived is a contextual unity. Most of what we do in the course of each day of our lives is non-reflective. This is not to say that our choices and actions are ignorant or antagonistic to reflection, but rather that much of what we do in the normal run of events is done without conscious thought. When activities are performed without conscious thought few if any distinctions, dichotomies, or separations pass before our awareness. While riding a bicycle, for example, I do not normally distinguish between myself and the bicycle. There is, of course, the felt resistance of the handlebars, pedals, and seat, but unless things go awry or unless I deliberately choose to reflect, the experience of the context of bicycle riding does not bring these notions to consciousness. Neither do we in the usual circumstances of riding a bicycle entertain the dichotomy of muscular versus mechanical motion or the separation of myself as a subject of sensation from the bicycle as cause of sensation. All of these divisions can be made, in a sense they are there to be made, and yet they are not made. One simply rides the bicycle with a felt sense of the unity of the whole experience at that moment and in that context. This sensed unity clears the mind; it makes it invisible or transparent to itself. The bicycle, the ride, and the rider are all as one.

It is this contextual unity which sets the stage for reflection. Conscious thought may begin because of a problem which bursts upon the scene and destroys the experienced unity, because of the sheer playfulness of a mind capable of rational division, or because the rider has a matured habit of reflection provoked and developed by the worlds of problem-solving, playfulness, or both. In any event, it is a characteristically human phenomenon that the contextual unity of our experience is periodically sundered by thought. Thought draws our attention to a part or parts of the contextual unity of an experience.

The essence of thought, then, is its ability to attend to parts of a whole experience in a way which, for the purposes at hand, allows it to ignore the essential unity of the situation in context. My thought of a sore muscle and its effect on the mechanical work of the bicycle effectively draws attention to a part of the experience while the whole unity of the ride is disguised. When my thought of this part ceases, a renewed unity of experience begins. This unity may itself be broken by thought and renewed at the end of that thought and so on. The challenge implicit in this ever changing relationship of unthinking experienced unity and thoughtful consciousness of part is the task of returning to a renewed unity of experience enriched by a latent consciousness of part. Perhaps I remember a minor injury to my muscle which resolves my concern, or I think of a treatment for the ache I will apply on my return from my ride. In either case and in the cases of a myriad of alternative scenarios, my consciousness becomes transparent to itself once again as I once again live through the unity of the bicycle riding context without conscious thought of part. This new unity, however, differs from the initial unity in some fashion because of the intervening conscious reflection. Perhaps my new experienced unity has a mood or a tone of concern or relief. Even if there is no perceptible difference in this new unity as lived, the second post-reflection unity is richer for the consciousness of part it has experienced; richer in the sense that it now contains more latent experience, memories, and intentions. This latent content may then be revived as a part of a conscious reflection in the future.

Reflection, then, is an awareness of parts isolated from an experienced whole. Its natural tendency seems to be to immerse itself into a whole once more, but a whole now enriched by latent consciousness of some parts of the whole. These parts may be of two quite different sorts.[2] I may think of my muscle as a part of my body just as I may consider the handlebars, pedals, and seat as parts of the bicycle. These kinds of parts might be called pieces or bits and conscious dwelling on them can give rise to a scientific consciousness. The knowledge of the various pieces of the body can lead to knowledge of medicine, anatomy, and ultimately to biochemistry. The knowledge of the various pieces of the bicycle can lead to knowledge of bicycle repair, mechanics, and ultimately to particle physics. There can be little doubt that the experienced sense of unity is enriched when the rider has the latent scientific consciousness of anatomy and mechanics. Such a latent consciousness is eminently useful both for the rider and the society he or she is part of. Not only is this latent conscious of obvious practical value but it is also satisfying in and of itself — a latent version of the pleasure of knowledge for its own sake. As humans we take delight in knowing and most of our knowing, at any given moment, is of this latent sort.

There is another sense of part, however, which can lead not to a scientific consciousness but to a philosophical consciousness. These parts are aspects or significances and, though they may really be parts of my experience, they can never exist separately the way that pieces can. I may think of my muscle ache as an aspect of an otherwise pleasurable experience or as a dimension of my bodily being, or as a sign of my age. All these thoughts may be parts of my conscious experience yet none of them refer to pieces in the same sense that my muscle is a separable bit of my body. I may equally consider the color, the weight, and the economy of my bicycle as aspects of my experience though here again none of these dimensions can stand alone as a piece. Though both are parts, aspects are fundamentally different from pieces.

The possibility of philosophical reflection relies on this human ability to draw out from the unity of lived experience various aspects or significances and to reintroduce them as latent elements of an enriched unity of consciousness. When they are drawn out by reflection these various aspects may be clarified in themselves, organized by being related to the whole or to other aspects, or criticized in light of some set of standards. I may, for example, clarify the economy of my bicycle by considering just how much money it cost and how much it saves. I may relate the weight of the bicycle to its design and to the materials of which it is made. I may criticize the bicycle's color by judging it against some standard of tastefulness. Thus philosophical reflection permits the clarification, organization, and critique of experience by the isolation and investigation of its aspects. When the fruits of such reflection are reintroduced into the renewed unity which follows, that renewed unity is enriched both practically and in itself. This reflection enriched unity of experience is latently wiser than before and is the source from which sound future decisions can issue.

In order to bring these insights closer to our concerns, let us consider the whole we call reality. Reality is the unity of all experienced unities. Surely no one of us has a complete grip on the fullness of reality but its essential unity is clear by contrast with what is admittedly unreal: dreams, illusions, hallucinations. For most of us, reality is clearly separated from these unreal worlds by the sense of wholeness it displays. Compared, for example, to the crazy quilt of our dreams, reality presents itself as orderly, con-

7

tinuous, and in harmony with itself. Indeed, most of the time, we do not consider the notion of reality at all since it is merely a name for the total experienced unity and coherence of everyday life. We live through reality and it is transparent to us as we do.

As it is the nature of philosophical reflection to isolate aspects of wholes, and as reality is one of the most important and all-encompassing wholes available to thought, one can expect that philosophical reflection will reveal important and pervasive aspects of reality. In fact, all great philosophers have done this in one way or another. It is not our task here to review the many aspects uncovered within reality by centuries of philosophy. Instead, let us examine this simple claim: Reality has two main aspects, the world of facts and the world of our human ideals. The dynamic interaction of facts and ideals constitutes our notion of reality.[3]

Initially it may seem implausible to include human ideals within the notion of reality. Ideals, after all, are not fulfilled in fact. There is a temptation to regard reality as coexistensive with the fact world; considering real all and only what is factually the case. But while the world of facts, what is the case in the world, must be an aspect of reality, facts themselves cannot be conceived without ideals. The very notion of a fact is a result of the impact of a human ideal. There are facts only when there is a consciousness that binds itself to the ideal of objectivity, when there are thinkers who attempt to impose impartiality on their thought. So far as we know, only human beings are capable of this attempt. Centuries of scientific assertions about facts and centuries of courts of law demanding "nothing but the facts" have lulled us into thinking that facts are "out there" independent of all human consciousness. Of course, there is some truth to this notion. A fact is what is independent of me and you. Facts are "hard" because they resist our desires and restrict our range of action. They are what science asserts and what fair court decisions are based on. But facts are not independent of all human thought. Though they may be "hard" in themselves, the knowing of facts requires more than feeling their resistance and restriction. Knowledge of fact requires reasoning and use of the many ideals contained without reasoning. Further, science and law are human activities, activities in which humans have imposed upon themselves the ideals of objectivity, impartiality, and proper methodology. Where is the fact in itself without some human consciousness to assert it, uncover it, and relate it systematically to other facts? The world of fact, the world as it is in itself without any human biases, is a creation of our collective human consciousness, a creation which other species seem incapable or uninterested in sharing with us. The world of fact is not fiction, yet it is not the whole of reality. It is only an aspect of the real, an aspect dependent to some extent on the world of human ideals.

On the other hand, it is a fact that humans have ideals. No factually accurate description of reality could do justice to our individual and collective experience if it did not admit the existence and importance of human ideals. We may tentatively define an ideal most broadly as any conceived state of affairs held to be admirable in itself by some agent. Ideals, as we have seen, help to make possible the world of fact by the imposition of standards of objectivity, standards taken to be practically valuable as well as admirable in themselves. Even more importantly, human ideals move individual persons and whole societies to action. Nothing is more revealing about a person or society or so valuable for predicting behavior than knowledge of the ideals which he, she, or they embrace.[4] To test this claim, consider the many ways you might describe yourself or your society and see which of these descriptions are primarily factual and which are primarily about ideals. This test should reveal how hard it is to conceive of an adequate description of any person or society which does not refer to some of the ideals which motivate them individually and collectively. Facts may establish the boundaries of human reality but ideals pervade that reality with significance and value. Ideals fill facts with meaning. They make life itself worth living by referring the facts of our lives to the goals and values we take to be worthy in themselves.

Futhermore, ideals have a dynamic relationship to reality which facts largely lack. The active assertion of an ideal can remake the fact world and reality with it. It is a matter of everyone's experience that character can be shaped in fact by the imposition of ideals. For example, by willful adherence to the ideal of honesty a person can become factually more honest. It is also a matter of our collective historical experience that ideals have remade the world of fact and have thus changed reality. For example, science, based on the ideal of objectivity, has paved the way for many powerful technologies which have changed facts. Social and political changes are also graphic evidences here. At one time, for example, the legal abolition of human slavery was an ideal held by a precious few people. Now, it is a fact. Such new historical realities are constantly being wrought out of the action of ideals on facts. An accurate accounting of the whole of reality would have to include these facts about ideals. Human persons live with their ideals in a world of fact and the dynamic interaction of the two constitutes what we call reality.

Philosophical reflection, by the isolation of our human ideals as aspects of the whole of reality, enables us to clarify, organize, and critique our ideals. Such reflection can improve our understanding and appreciation of our ideals both in their relationships to one another and in their relationships to the whole of reality. If an ideal is what is held to be admirable in itself, then the acts of clarifying, organizing, and criticizing our ideals can result in greater appreciation of them, replacement of them with ideals taken to be more admirable, or both. This activity can thus enhance the attractiveness of ideals to the reflective agent by making the agent more aware of ideals and by making the ideals more admirable in themselves. Because of the natural tendency for reflective consciousness to return to enrich the lived unity from which it has isolated these aspects and because it is from this enriched unity of reality that concrete human decisions and actions emerge, philosophy can help us remake reality and remake it so as

9

to conform more nearly to our ideals. Not only is this a description of philosophical reflection; it is also a formula for human progress. The theoretical activity of philosophy is thus eminently practical because it helps us to idealize the fact world; it helps us to make reality better.

C. Truth: Of Facts and Ideals

It is appropriate in light of our discussion of reality to raise the question of truth since the most rudimentary insight about truth is that it is what adequately describes reality. A true description of an event, for instance, describes the various elements of the event and their relationships one to another as they really did occur. Truth, one might say, is the faithful expression of the real and the real is the object that truth seeks to faithfully express. What are the implications of this sketch of a theory of reality for the question of truth?

If we begin with the world of fact as an aspect of reality, our answer appears straightforward. The expression of a fact, if it really is a fact, just is the truth. One could conceive of individual facts as the pieces of the fact world, itself an aspect of reality. As we have seen, examination of pieces give rise to a scientific consciousness. Consequently, facts will have a special role in the project of science as the human activity of uncovering the fact world. The goal of natural science is the faithful description of the fact world and its various factual pieces.

As simple as this sounds, the situation becomes more complex when one considers the project of science as an historical activity of human beings.[5] What once was considered fact and its expression true has often been overturned by later scientific work. Once it was taken as fact and its assertion as true that the earth was the center of the motion of all heavenly bodies. Once it was taken as fact and its assertion as true that the atom was indivisible, and that time and space provide an absolute framework for all events. These examples could be multiplied to include every significant advance in scientific knowledge. As new fact replaces old fact, old truth becomes false in the light of new truth. One can reasonably expect that so long as science as we know it continues to advance, such adjustments in fact and truth will continue apace. Thus at any point in human history short of the end of science itself, what constitutes a fact and its expression a truth will have to be considered to be tentative and open to future adjustment. There may be times when we will have to act as if we know these facts to be wholly true, but on reflection we will know that we do not have sufficient intellectual basis for the confidence demanded by action.[6] The fact I must act on today may tomorrow be no fact at all.

Also we know that scientists do not merely describe series of individual facts but that they knit these facts together into larger scientific theories.[7] At any point in its development, a scientific theory will contain some very well confirmed facts, some less well confirmed facts, and some highly speculative guesses about other facts. Since even the very well confirmed facts may be overturned by future advance, a scientific theory is always quite tentative in principle (though one can recognize vast differences of degree in the tentativeness of theories depending upon the preponderance of well confirmed facts). So while it is true that scientific theories give facts a larger framework and thus greater explanatory power, they do so by introducing more doubt in principle about the facts alleged by the theory. As difficult as it is in principle to be sure that any given fact may be relied on to continue to prove true as science advances, it is that much more difficult to be sure that scientific theories will continue to prove true. Only a century ago, for example, it was thought that Newtonian physical theory was final and true. Now it has been superceded by relativity theory and by the theories of quantum mechanics.

Finally, we now know that the fact world, while it appears to be relatively stable to the eye of common sense, is in a process of change itself. Nature has evolved and continues to evolve. This physical evolution opens the possibility that even when science has established some fact as adequately as it can, the fact itself may change. A simple example of this is gross geological change on the earth's surface: volcanoes, earthquakes, erosion, etc. Even such an obvious fact as the existence of an island may be a fact only for some limited time period. A more profound possibility here is that the very laws of nature, the laws with which other facts are organized and explained, may themselves be slowly evolving.[8]

Let us draw these points together. Even in the easiest case of defining truth, that of natural scientists' descriptions of pieces of the fact world; even here, we find the truth of an assertion to be tentative and open to future adjustment. The changes in what are considered facts, the change in theories to organize facts and suspected facts, and the changes within the fact world itself combine to suggest humility in asserting the definitive truth of any description of the fact world. This point is even more graphic when applied to the human sciences. Here few facts are well confirmed, competing theories proliferate, and the object of knowledge is elusive; human beings changing dramatically in some respects, and especially when aware of being observed.

Perhaps the best way to salvage a theory of truth in such circumstances would be to say this. First, truth does mean the faithful expression of reality and, in this case, of a fact. Secondly, at any given time in human history we shall have to be content to regard our "truths" as incomplete, partial, and subject to future revision — even in cases where we have no practical alternative to acting as if they were fully true. Finally, we can hope, change within the fact world itself aside, that continued scientific inquiry, will tend to establish an increasingly stable set of facts and truths about them. In other words, we can hope that human commitment to the indefinitely continued discipline of the ideal of objectivity will tend to correct the errors contained within any stage of science and will tend to converge our beliefs toward what is really true. This is no more nor less than to say that it is reasonable to hope that our species can learn from its collective experience. Even with respect to change within the fact world, it may be reasonable to hope for an increasingly stable set of truths about changing facts so that we can include in the fact world facts about the change of facts, for example, facts about the cause and results of volcanoes. This may not be the neat and simple theory of truth from which common sense begins, but it is one honest to the human activity of science and to the fallibility evident in its history.

When we turn to the other aspect of reality, to the world of human ideals, the situation is quite different. If truth is the faithful expression of reality and ideals are an aspect of reality, the world of ideals will have to figure in our consideration of truth as well. A first point is the obvious: It is true that humans as individuals and in societies have ideals which motivate their conduct. A true description of any human event, a war for example, would have to describe not only the facts of the case (battles, victories, defeats) but also the conceived states of affairs taken to be admirable in themselves by the participants (ideals of patriotism, defense of culture, restoration of homelands) and how these ideals motivated the participants in the event. Accounts omitting these facts about ideals could not possibly be true.

If we look to those disciplines which study ideals, those whose concentration on this aspect of reality develops a philosophical consciousness such as the humanities and the human sciences; if we look to these disciplines, we will find the same difficulties noted above and more difficulties peculiar to ideals. There is wide disagreement among humanists and those in the human sciences as to what factually were or are the specific ideals of any person or culture at any time.[9] This situation, of course, mirrors the ambiguities embedded in the relationship between ideals and human motivation. We are often confused and only half aware of the ideals which motivate us in any case and the conflicts between them in some cases can be both deeply felt and hard to articulate. Ideals are compelling but they are inherently vague. Not only, then, do the descriptions of ideals change through time as descriptions of the fact world do, but there is also a wide array of conflicting descriptions of the ideals of a person or a society being urged at any given time.

Also, as facts are organized into theories, so ideals tend to be knit together to form whole ideal worldviews of persons and societies. A description of any individual or collective worldview of ideals is frought with all the difficulties of validating scientific theories plus the ambiguities inherent to ideals themselves. As scientific theories will inevitably contain some weakly confirmed claims about facts, so descriptions of whole worldviews will inevitably contain some weakly confirmed claims about ideals. And again, the ideals themselves are vague. Further, it appears altogether possible for persons and cultures to have worldviews whose ideals are in tension with one another or are outright incompatible. One need think here only of the long association of Christianity and slavery to make this point.

Finally, while we have had to admit some measure of change in the fact world due to physical evolution, we shall have to admit a far more wholesale change in the ideal world due to cultural evolution. Simply consider the cultural contexts which provided for the ideals of the ancient Greek aristocrat, of the medieval saint, of the modern imperialist, of the contemporary individual.[10] As societies have evolved so have the ideals and worldviews of persons in those societies. This point suggests a sort of reliance of ideals on facts. As the facts of a society change, ideals too have changed. One can justly reverse this point as well — as persons have changed their ideals so have they factually changed their societies. These changed facts may then allow for the development of new ideals, themselves changing the facts again, and so on. Can we meaningfully speak of truth in such a changing situation?

We can clarify and restate this question in terms of a long-standing philosophical problem, viz., the relationship between what is and what ought to be, a distinction which fairly mirrors our distinction between the fact world and the ideal world.[11] The fact world tells us what is, but the world of ideals, since it motivates action, tells us what ought to be. To restate our question in these terms, can we ever meaningfully assert the truth of what ought to be? In light of what we have already seen, any affirmative answer will have to be at least as tentative as the assertion of factual truth and then more so because of the ambiguity and vagueness of human ideals. Nevertheless, it is a fact and true that persons and societies have ideals and that these ideals motivate their actions. These ideals are born not only out of changing cultural situations, but also out of the possibilities inherent in the very nature of human persons and human communities. The ideal of honesty, for example, while it takes very different expressions in the hands of different ages and cultures, appears to be an ideal implicit in the very nature of the human person's ability to communicate to another and to freely choose to do so with an intent of truthfulness or deceit. The ideal of persons caring for one another seems to be implicit in the frailities of each individual person's existence and in the emotive bonding of human communities. If this is so, that is, if some ideals reach across many or even all differing factual circumstances, then reflection should reveal these ideals to be the most compelling to us. Clarification, organization, and critique of these ideals should make them appear to be the best ideals we can choose to motivate our actions. Perhaps then we can say that these ideals truly ought to be. Which ideals these are and how they relate one to another is a question for ongoing humanities and human sciences discussion and for personal and social choice.

Let us draw this discussion together with a strategy analogous to that used with the fact world. First, truth in this context can mean two things, what ideals are factually held by persons and societies and what ideals ought to be held. Secondly, factual descriptions of ideals and normative assertions of which ideals ought to be held must be regarded as most tentative "truths", as incomplete, partial, and subject to future revision —

13

again even where we have no practical alternative to acting as if they were fully true. Finally, we can hope that the indefinitely continued study of ideals under the self-imposed standard of intersubjectivity, if not objectivity, of the humanities and the human sciences, will tend to establish an increasingly stable set of facts about ideals. Here this hope is more attenuated by the inherent ambiguity and vagueness of the ideal world than is the analogous hope for the convergence of truths about the fact world. This is especially so in the case of the normative assertion that it is true that this or that ideal is one we ought to embrace. Given the ambiguities already described and given the fact that the acceptance of an ideal as normative involves a choice (though often unconsciously so), it will be hard to ever feel confident in principle with the assertion that any given ideal ought to be embraced as definitively true.

In spite of these admissions, we constantly act on our ideals and in doing so express an implied faith that they are true ideals, or at least the best ideals available to us. Furthermore, if ideals have the reconstructive character suggested above, that is, if action based upon an ideal can alter both the fact world and other aspects of the ideal world, then ideals can alter reality in a way which brings reality into greater conformity with the ideal. Thus there is a sense in which ideals can, if earnestly acted upon, literally make themselves true.[12] There is then a hope allowed by this process: that the most compelling ideals we embrace now will continue to be embraced by agents of good will into the indefinite future and that the collective weight of these ideal commitments and the factual changes made by the actions they direct will tend to remake reality in their image. Thus we can hope that our ideals will make themselves true. The strategy that suggests itself for agents in the middle of this process, as we all are, is to reflectively embrace the best ideals offered by our culture and circumstances and to assert them into the future with intellectual humility but with practical vigor. What are the best ideals available is a matter for continuous intelligent debate and the vigor with which we assert them must be moderated by a humility born from the sincere admission that we may be wrong ultimately. Nevertheless, reality demands that we act, our ideals are the bases upon which we act, and we must act as if our ideals are the true ones, the ones towards which the indefinite extension of earnest human reflection and action will tend to converge.

Chapter 2.

Rational Animals

A. Nature and the Emotions

Now that we have given some flesh to the notion of an ideal and to its relationship to fact, reality, and truth, we can turn to a consideration of the ideals available to us in this culture at this time. Specifically, let us consider the traditional ideal of the human person as a rational animal and the meaning such an ideal can have for us today.[1] Let us consider the wider notion first, viz., our being as animals.

Traditionally, our animal nature was held to be the repository of all things nonrational, especially the body and its multiple natural abilities such as growth, healing, ability to take on habits of behavior, etc. Our animal nature was also thought to be the source of our emotional life at least so far as the emotions were taken to be raw passions, feelings wholly unmediated by reason. It is important to note at the outset that this animal dimension of our lives is not irrational but nonrational. Irrationality is a failure in a being or an aspect of a being, a failure to be the rational being it is or could be. It is no failure to be nonrational. As we do not fault dogs for being irrational, neither should we fault our bodies nor our passions.

In fact, the nonrational character of our bodies and passions is an important benefit both to our rational selves and to our entire being as persons. Rationality, as we have seen, requires the conscious interruption of the lived unity of experience, attention to part of an experience, and, if ideals are the parts at stake, decision and action based on those ideals. All of this takes time, control, and is marked throughout by the changing and provisional character of the search for truth. Even the most conscientious of reasonings is slow, delicate, and open to error. Consequently, it is a great liberation that our bodies and passions work by themselves without need for conscious thought. Were persons to rationally think through their growth, healing, and ability to form habits, one could expect that our hold on life itself would be far more tenuous than it is. Were each of us to rationally fashion our fundamental passions, one could expect that our hold on our mental balance would be far more tenuous than it is. We can be properly grateful for the nonrational aspects of our persons.

The human body comes to each of us initially as a natural fact, a given. The union of our parents' germ cells establishes a genetic blueprint for growth and development in gestation and for a host of further developments after birth. The conduct of life after conception is a subtle and perhaps inextricable weaving of genetic and environmental factors. Our genetic inheritance establishes certain facts and possibilities for our bodily and mental developments, and the course of life's stimuli and choices confirm and elaborate those facts and select among those possibilities.

In spite of this appearance of a given genetic structure and the happenstances of life for each of us, we know scientifically that DNA itself is not simply a given but has itself evolved in interaction with the environment. In evolutionary terms, our species' DNA represents the most highly adaptive stage of generations of trial, error, and success in the passing on of genetic information. Our genetic inheritance comes to us then as a sedimentation of genetic and environmental factors, a concrete expression of centuries of interaction between somatic information and extrasomatic circumstances. One might think of our genes as the physical memory of generations of human and prehuman experience.

Our passions are also due to our bodily animal selves. For the sake of clarity on this point, let us stipulate a distinction between passions and emotions. Passions, on this account, are the raw, unmediated feelings of life, the spontaneous affective reactions to experience. We are born with a natural energy of the passions. In all likelihood the basic passions have a survival value related to our animal ability to feel pleasure and pain. Desire for food and affection, fear of assault, anger at frustration; these and other basic passions have an obvious utility to members of a species in a dangerous natural and social environment. As the name suggests, passions are what we are passive to; passions overcome us, carry us away, place us beside ourselves.

Emotions, by contrast, while still affective, are mediated to some extent by reason. The emotion of satisfaction at a job well done, or the emotion of concern for the destiny of the human race, or the emotion of fear of a plane crash; all these are emotions which have been shaped considerably by conscious thought. Emotion can be thought of here as the result of the interaction of passion and active reasoning. It is a commonplace of life, for example, that reasoning and facts brought to light through reasoning can alter the emotions. One no longer resents a snub discovered to be inadvertent. One no longer despises an accused individual exhonorated of the crime. It is also a fact of common experience that emotions can be rational or irrational, that is, that some emotions can be inappropriate. Exaggerated fear of cancer in a young and healthy individual or a feeling of anger toward an innocent person are inappropriate and irrational emotions. Finally, it is also a fact that our emotional lives can be educated and refined. Acquired tastes for theatre, literature, and gourmet foods are common examples. Less obvious is the fact that our specifically moral emotions are also products of education. Repugnance at the cruelty of one person to another is a learned emotion, as is the feeling of disappointment in an unfulfilled promise, and wholehearted joy in the success of another. Such moral emotions are drawn out of our passions through education and reflection on experience.[2]

16

If we place this observation about our emotional life in a larger historical context, we can see that culture generally is the great educator of the emotions. Our emotions are shaped by the traditional stories, songs and literature, and even the humor of our culture. With the advent of the mass media and its ability to affect the emotional lives of millions at once and in a graphic fashion, this point becomes plainer than ever. Our cultures help to fashion our native passions into conventional emotions. And since the masses of people respond to their environment primarily at the emotive level, the power of a culture to shape events is awesome indeed.

Just as our DNA can be regarded at the physical sedimentation of generations of interaction between genes and experience, so our cultures can be thought of as the social sedimentation of generations of interaction between our native passions and our conscious reasoning. The emotive life of one generation begins with the achievement of rational interaction with the passions of the generations preceding and affecting it. Similarly, the emotive attainment of generations of future persons will be built upon the accumulated emotional experience implicit in today's culture and in those to follow. The emotive lives of persons and cultures are continually reconstructing themselves in light of passions and reasonings about new facts in human history and new or clarified ideals. It has taken, for example, significant changes in the facts of human history to bring about the emotion of fear of nuclear annihilation. It has taken significant changes in human ideals to bring about emotional attachment to the peace and well-being of persons of all nations into the indefinite future.

The connection here suggested between emotions and ideals is crucial. If ideals are those conceived states of affairs taken to be so admirable in themselves that they are capable of moving us to act to realize them in greater part, then our reaction to ideals must have a powerful emotive component. It is not through reasoning alone that persons and cultures commit themselves to great present sacrifices for future goods. Nor is it due to the power of raw passion. It is through the mediation of reason and passion in the educated emotions of persons and cultures that we are driven to embrace ideals. Our ideals move us by attraction. We desire to see them realized, if not fully, then at least in greater part. The desire to realize ideals in fact is one of the most fundamental of the emotions and one capable of great consequences for human action.

For those who are concerned to promote the realization of the best ideals available to us at this time and in this culture, there is a clear implication in these observations. Whatever these ideals are, they cannot be promoted and defended by reasoning alone. Instead they must become more fully embedded into the spontaneous emotional responses of persons in our culture. If, for example, we are concerned to promote the ideal of human solidarity across national boundaries, then persons of the present and the future must be educated to feel good about instances of international cooperation and to feel bad about cases of jingoism. This feeling good and feeling bad must pervade our traditional stories, songs and literature, humor, and radio and television programs if we want this ideal to be a real force in the lives of most people. There is always a thin line between education and indoctrination when one speaks of emotional education and the boundary between these two must be respected in a free society. Still, if we ignore the force of the connection between our ideals and the evolving emotional life of our culture, reasoning alone will not sustain our ideals.

Even if the clarification, organization, and criticism of reasoning could sustain our ideals, one still must admit the great emotive force within reasoning itself. Clarification of a concept sorts out the emotions as well as the cognitions involved. Rational organization itself is strongly related to a powerful emotional repugnance at inconsistency and contradiction. Criticism must have standards and reasoning cannot indefinitely supply reasons for the selection of these standards, and then reasons for the selection of standards for the selection of standards, etc. A critical investigation does not stop when we reach the reasons for the standards of the standards of the standards and so on. Instead, specific criticism of any sort stops when we are emotionally satisfied, when we feel that enough reasons have been supplied in this context to silence our questions and to satisfy our wonder.[3] Even the very commitment to the use of reasoning where appropriate has its emotional dimension: we are uncomfortable with pure guess work and outraged by stupidity. In short, reasoning in general and in its parts is intertwined with emotions.

Thus our animal self is a critically important part of our being and is not to be demeaned by comparison with reason. The evolution of our animal body has produced our brains and thus has made reasoning of any kind possible. Our emotional life gives depth and efficacy to reason by uniting it with the power of raw passions. Achievements in the realization of human ideals are made, carried, and built upon from generation to generation largely by emotional attractions and repugnances. Our animal self is thus a central and precious part of what we are and can become as human persons.

B. Reason and Freedom

When we consider the human person as a rational animal, this is not meant to exclude other critically important dimensions of our experience, as is clear from our discussion on the significance of the body and the emotions. The addition of the modifier 'rational' is meant to point out a uniqueness of our species that goes beyond what is found throughout the remainder of the animal kingdom. We are the animals that reason and we display this ability in the complexities of our languages and behaviors and in the characters of the persons and societies we create. We are not, it hardly needs to be said, completely rational at all times, nor is it clear that this would be a wholly desirable state of affairs were it even possible. Instead the human person is a whole unity of many inheritances and capacities; reason is an aspect of this unity of our being. We do reason; but we do not have a piece which is a rational self or a mind separate from our bodies. This is a fact available to all.[4] Reason expresses itself in a conscious fashion episodically and as interwoven within the larger fabric of our feelings and habits.

Reasoning, or the ability to reflect upon experience, is itself composed of the abilities to clarify an experience, organize it, and critique it. Reason clarifies by its primary operation of attending to parts of an otherwise unitary experience. This attention to parts of a whole can result in an enriched consciousness, one that "sees" more in its experience. This increase in mental vision is graphic in the comparison between an expert and a novice in nearly any human endeavor. The expert is such because of an enhanced ability to perceive, because of a learned skill of finding more hints, implications, and possibilities in a situation. The expert carpenter, for example, immediately identifies the specific tools needed for a task; the expert mathematician straightaway sees the strategy that must be followed for a solution to a problem; the expert musician perceives the possibilities in an auditory experience. In all of these cases, the unclarified experience of the novice is stunned by the remarkable perspicuity of the expert. Yet this seeing, as hard as it may be to teach directly, is clearly a learned skill and is at the heart of the education which passes one from novice to expert in any field. Of course, this is, as we say, a matter of experience, but it is experience consciously strained by the effort to see more, by the observance of significant part, by the self discipline of serious attention. It is a matter of experience reflected upon.

Not only are we capable of such an increase in clarity of mental vision through reasoning, but we are also able to organize. The various parts of a whole generally will have multiple relationships among themselves, to the whole, and to other wholes. Reasoning explores these relationships by drawing out implications, ordering and categorizing, and systematizing. This is the source of mathematics, logic, and all theory construction. Human reason contains both a descriptive and creative expression of this ability. We are able to discover relationships within a given whole and to faithfully follow the facts in an articulation of these relationships. The discovery of the basic chemical elements and their organization into atomic weight, number, etc. is a case in point. On the other hand, this same ability allows us to create and impose an order on what may not have even been a unitary whole at all but for this operation of reason. The construction of the rules of a game, design of a new building, planning for one's future; each of these are cases of human creation and imposition of organization. One of the great difficulties with any theory of truth is suggested here. It is often very hard to know in any concrete case how much of the organization we impute to a situation is discovered to be there and how much is (unconsciously) created and imposed by our reasoning ability. Restated in terms we have already used, it is often hard to know how much organization is part of the fact world and how much is part of our ideal world.

The last dimension of reasoning is our ability to critique experience. Criticism in philosophy does not imply a negative stance as it does in common parlance. Here criticism means the search for justification and validation. Not only may I clarify and organize the content of an experience, but I may also find it acceptable, unacceptable, or some subtle combination of both. For example, after perceiving the possibility of constructing a new building and after organizing its design, I might well reject the result as unacceptable. The acceptability of an experience must be appraised by comparison with some standards. The choice of such standards must itself be justified, but typically these standards may be found in one of two ways. The acceptability of some situation may be judged in terms of standards implicit in the situation itself. For example, I may judge that the building I have designed is not adequate to the conceived building I had anticipated at the outset. Or I may find that given the limitations on my resources, I can not afford to build a structure close enough to the standards I set out with. On the other hand, my design may be unacceptable because of standards imposed from without the situation: by municipal building codes, by a general lack of sufficient resources, or by my judgement that there are other, more significant activities for my time and energies. The questions of the location of the proper standards and the adequacy of their use in any given case are complex and the source of much human controversy from the construction of buildings to the construction of societies. Nevertheless, criticism is a distinctly human capacity and one which allows for improvement in our condition through the reflective embrace of the acceptable and the reflective rejection of the unacceptable.

If reasoning begins by the reflective isolation of parts of our experienced whole, it often terminates in an act of will. Will, like our emotions and reasonings, is not a separate piece of our minds or bodies but that aspect of our whole being which permits us to form intentions to act and to carry intentions into action. The act of will is at the heart of human choice. Except in those activities in which we recognize the need for the exercise of thought for its own sake as in pure science, contemplative thought, or in mental play; except in such cases, reasoning is eminently practical since it terminates in an act of will. Acts of will pervade our experience as we each moment choose our activities and even the positions of our bodies. Yet most of these acts of will are unconscious choices. These choices, the vast majority of those we make, are carried by our emotional life and by our fixed habits of choice making. They are like the habitual morning cup of coffee — a choice to be sure, but a choice long since become feeling and habit and thus unconscious. Reason is practical when it precedes and informs an act of will, when it makes a choice conscious and reflective.

Thus reasoning, one of our distinctive species characteristics, leads us directly to another specifically human experience: freedom. Reasoning can make us free. If what has been said above about the cultural formation of our emotional life is accurate and if these emotions give rise to actions which become habitual and unreflective, then most of what we do as persons is unfree. We do make choices, of course; brewing and drinking coffee, for example, requires a host of choices. But these choices are unconscious and evolved from a culturally formed desire for coffee, a desire whose satisfaction time and again has fixed a habit of behavior. Have I really made a free choice to have coffee this morning? Hardly. But I can if I reason. If, for example, it were to occur to me that I drink too much coffee, that it is too expensive or hazardous to my health, my next cup may well be preceded by conscious reflection and a deliberate act of will. I then freely choose to have or not to have coffee. This choice will follow a process of reflection, a process of clarifying what is at stake, organizing it with other considerations, and criticizing it in light of some standards; in this case those of finances, health, or both.

The rational and free choices of persons become facts. These facts are integrated into the web of the life of the emotions and they establish tendencies to make such choices again, tendencies to take on habits. Emotions and habits, therefore, set the context for the possibility of rational and free choice and carry the results of such choices unconsciously beyond themselves into the future. Gradually, reason and freedom come to be more fully integrated into emotions and habits and come to make even unconscious choices more fully embody reason and freedom. The self-consciously rational and free choice of a career, for example, is embodied in the lifetime of career related emotions and habits which follow. On a larger scale, whole societies can liberate themselves from the emotions and habits they have inherited by the accumulated impact of individual rational and free choices and the resultant establishment of new or altered emotions and social habits.

It must be added here that in both cases, of the individual person and of the whole of society, reason and freedom are relative and contextual. No person or society is absolutely reasonable or absolutely free in all situations, whatever that might even mean. Instead, reasoning and thus freedom arise against a unified background of received emotions, habits, facts, and ideals and they resolve themselves back into this unity once again. Reason and freedom are thus episodic in the totality of human life. Nevertheless, these can be important, self-defining episodes as they can make the new unity of experience a bit more latently reasonable and free. Futhermore, it seems clear that frequent episodes of rational choice can develop a positive affective stance toward reasoning and choosing freely and that rational choice can itself become a habit, a habit of transcending habit. Thus reason and freedom both stand apart from and enter into the world of emotion and habit.

There is one powerful objection to this view that must be acknowledged. Some have claimed that all human action is unfree, that it is all determined by past events.[5] These past events typically include our genetic structure, psychological conditioning, socio-economic position, etc. There can be no denying the power of the rational argument that can be constructed to show that at root all human choice is determined and unfree. There is only one reply which can be made and, however inadequate it may sound, it must be made. Free choice on the basis of conscious reflection is a fact of our personal experience.[6] However difficult it may be to reconcile this experience with our ever increasing knowledge of the causal sources of human behavior, it remains a fact of experience. This experience is most graphic in cases of serious conflict in reflection and choice, as in the case of choosing between two very bad alternatives. It is also graphic in the case of temptation, when one feels poised between what one wants and what one ought to do. These experiences and others like them which reveal rational choice in the concrete are far too intimate a part of our lives to dismiss as insignificant or illusory. As a matter of fact, we experience ourselves as capable of rational and free choice. As a matter of ideal, we find ourselves capable of conceiving ourselves as potentially rational and free beings. This is implied in our notion of what it is to be a person. Without this conviction, the prospect of progress inherent in our ability to make our own lives and our societies more rational and more free would be lost.

C. Transcendence

The human ability to clarify, organize, and critique the received experience of emotion and habit enables persons and societies to move beyond themselves and their situations. This is a fundamental fact about human beings: We are capable of transcending ourselves.

This point has already been suggested in our discussion of our body and culture. Our genetic inheritance represents the result of generations of successful physical transcendence. Physical evolution can be understood as the natural world's ability to go beyond any present forms of life to other more adaptive forms. Although biologists are rightfully loathe as scientists to speak of progress in evolution, from the point of view of our own species, there can be no doubt that physical evolution has been, and therefore can be, progressive. Presumably we evolved from forms of life not unlike the other animal species now extant, species lacking the higher mental functions central to our existence. It is not arrogance nor a denial of our animal nature to assert the obvious, viz., that our nature is superior to the rest of the animal kingdom with respect to the characteristics we most value, with respect to all the higher mental functions made possible by the size and organization of our brain. As this is better than the capacities of other animals and is the result of evolution, the conclusion that physical evolution has been progressive in one straightforward sense is unavoidable. The very body of the human person represents nature's own transcendence of prior limitations.

These higher mental functions themselves allow for an ongoing self-transcendence by our species. Unlike the case of other animals whose access to stored information is largely genetic, human beings can store information outside the body. The nest building abilities of birds, for example, is a highly complex set of behaviors evolved over centuries and passed on to each individual bird in the genetic information it receives at conception. Though some animals can learn from experience directly in their own individual lifetimes, for the most part the learning of animals from experience is a species property contained within their genetic structure. It is thus generally slow to change; it is inherently conservative. By contrast, humans can learn a great deal from experience individually over and above the information received genetically, and this new learning can be stored and passed on to others outside the body. The first human to fashion a wheel as a tool, for example, added significant information to our species and passed this information on to others in an extrasomatic fashion, through example, gesture, speech, etc. With the advent of relatively stable written languages, of libraries, radio, television, computers, and of social institutions created and sustained specifically to foster the systematic advance of learning in both theoretical and practical realms, our species has transcended the informational limitations of genetic inheritance. Information can now be rapidly accumulated, widely shared, and securely stored outside the human body. Information for us is now inherently dynamic; we are continually transcending the learning we have received.

Human beings also transcend themselves in their time consciousness, another characteristic largely lacking in other animals. Because of our ability to conceptualize time, we are always free to transcend the present by attention to the future or by revery in the past. This ability to place the present moment within the larger framework of expected future and remembered past allows us to transcend the attractions, griefs, and demands of the moment through an imaginative relocation of ourselves in time. Without this ability to go beyond the present our notion of self-identity and our ability to defer present satisfactions for future benefits would be diminished or destroyed. A similar if weaker point can be made about space — through imagination we can relocate ourselves and thus transcend in part the limitations of present space. As animals with bodies we are here and now, but as rational animals who think, plan, and remember we can transcend this limitation to be there and then.

Another graphic example of the self-transcendence of the human person is that unique combination of emotions and reflections we call curiosity. While other species do display a similar characteristic, the curiosity of animals is but a pale and ineffectual shadow of this compelling and consuming dimension of our lives. From the nearly empty convention of asking another "what's new?" to the questions that lay at the very edge of scientific research, humans are driven by a need to know more, to discover more, to satisfy the urge of curiosity. There appears to be no natural nor conventional limits to the range and power of human curiosity. It is at the heart of the popularity of newspapers and television as well as at the heart of the commitment of the scientist. Curiosity always seeks to know what it does not know, to go beyond its own state of knowing. It can be an amusing friend or an oppressive master, but always it is insatiable and self-transcending. It is curiosity that is the mainspring of our drive to know the world of fact.

There is also a self-trascending character to human creativity. We are driven by our natures not only to know but also to make, express, create. From the great works of fine art, to the redecoration of a living room, to the design of a new machine, to the plans for a new city, humans are creating and recreating their environment. Here again there appears to be no natural nor conventional limits to this human creativity. Constantly, there are new artistic movements, new mechanical inventions, new social institutions, new fashions in housing, dress, and play. Creation builds on creation without apparent loss of ideas or energy. What is once made is remade and then made again, each generation incorporating its own new styles, new inventions, and new possibilities for future creation.

Just as it is curiosity which binds us to the fact-world, it is creativity that drives us to the world of ideals. Ideals are not only patterns for creative action but they are themselves subject to creation and recreation. As a state of affairs taken to be admirable in itself, an ideal can be clarified to enhance its attractiveness, organized with other ideals to insure its consistency, and judged acceptable by reflection. When this is done, the will can embrace it wholeheartedly and recreate portions of reality to more fully realize the ideal in fact. But this changes the facts and creates a new reality, a new whole whose own implied ideals need clarification, organization and critique. The repetition of this process can generate new ideals or new versions of old ideals. Again, this is self-transcendence. And again, there is the possibility of progress inherent in this process. If reality can be made over in part to conform to what is ideal and ideals themselves can be continually reformulated to be clearer, more consistent, and more acceptable, then the character of reality can be made more ideal and our ideals can be made more real. It would be too much to claim that such a process of improvement is inevitable. The resistance of the fact world is too strong and our grasp on the direction and successes of this procession of ideals is too weak for such a confidence. Nevertheless, this process of self-transcending advance clearly occurs on some occasions and may well be occuring on many other occasions. Most importantly, it seems to be within the realm of our human abilities to choose personally and socially that such a self-transcending advance be a part of all occasions in which serious and deeply felt human ideals are at stake.

Another way to put this point is by reference to the notion of perfection. An ideal is as attractive as it is to us no doubt because it represents in thought the perfection of some aspect of reality, the fulfillment of a felt possibility, the mental development into excellence of what is now only good. The fact that ideals are so central to our human existence is an expression of the force of the notion of perfection in our consciousness.[7] As persons and as a species, we are seldom satisfied with what is partial and only good but seek fullness and excellence. The only goal finally acceptable to our insatiable curiosity is complete omniscience. The only goal finally acceptable to our manifold creativity is complete onmipotence. In this sense, then, the tug of perfection structured into our ideals inevitably makes human beings God seekers since the attractiveness of these many kinds of perfection could only be wholly satisfied by the All-Perfect.[8] And just as inevitably our ideals will be a constant source of frustration and unhappiness, since we are driven to seek what cannot be fully had within the constraints of the world of fact.

But even in this poignant if not absurd situation, our ideals as human persons are critical and valuable parts of our reality. If we cannot have perfection in the fact world, at least we can have the task of continually perfecting the fact world through our ideals. In this manner, we can continue to transcend ourselves as persons and as societies. Perhaps it is our human destiny to participate in the perfecting process of the All-Perfect through the progressive realization of our ideals in the world of fact.[9] But whatever our final destiny may be, in our somatic and extra-somatic learnings, in our consciousness of time and space, in our curiosity and creativity, and in our vague but powerful ideals of perfection, a fact of the human person and human societies is self-transcendence.

Not only are our ideals instrumental in this self-transcendence, but self-transcendence may itself be applied to our ideals and thus open up to us another ideal, an ideal of ideals, a consummate ideal: the ideal of human persons and human societies indefinitely transcending and perfecting themselves. In other words, our very having of ideals at all suggests the possibility of ideals in our dealings with the ideal, a self-transcendence in the creation of ideals. The most obvious way of providing some context to this notion is with reference to ourselves and our societies. As we are capable of creating and acting on personal ideals, so we are capable of creating and acting on the ideal of each human person continually creating and acting on ideals through free and reasonable personal choices. As we are capable of creating and acting on social ideals, so we are capable of creating and acting on the ideal of each society continually creating and acting on ideals through free and reasonable social choices. In simpler terms, the self-transcendence of ideals suggests the ideals of self-transcending persons in self-transcending societies. Concretely, the factual expression of these ideals would yield autonomous human persons in progressive human societies. Elaboration of this point will require further investigation of the person and society, of the self and its social dimensions.

Chapter 3.

The Self and Society

A. The Self Alone

The theory of reality sketched above underscores the centrality of ideals both in our conception of reality and in our active reconstruction of reality through the use of our ideals as guides for actions. There are many ideals available to persons in our society at our time. As aspects of reality, ideals will be constitutive of virtually all human activities; where there is human reality, there will also be human ideals. Because of this pervasive character of ideals, it cannot be our task here to catalogue them all, even if such a task is possible. Nor it is part of this project to compare the acceptability of ideals against some external standard, as important a philosophical task as that might be. Our task is ultimately the practical one of applying an ideal or constellation of closely related ideals to concrete factual situations in contemporary medical care contexts. Since this task is practical, it involves an act of will, a conscious choice to embrace an ideal and to draw out its implications for action. The selection of ideals, therefore, is a free choice. Ideals other than those chosen here can be similarly elaborated for the sake of application to practice and, of course. But if our choice, admittedly free, is also to be rational, there must be some reasons for the selection of one or some ideals rather than others. These reasons, like all reasons, will be contextual and related to the current state of ideals available in a real sense to our culture at this time and to the factual basis for their realization in our current emotions and habits. The conclusions reached above about our natures as rational and free beings and about the ideal of ideals in our discussion of transcendence suggests reasons in the ideal for choosing the ideals of autonomous human persons in progressive human societies. Embrace of these ideals would affirm our abilities to be rational and free. It would also preserve and foster our self-transcending process of creating and applying ideals and thus would underscore the significance of this peculiarly human ability. It is also a fact that many human societies, especially those societies identifying with the culture of the democracies of the West, have reached something of a consensus in the feelings and habits embodied in their religions, laws, social conventions and personal consciences, a consensus to accept in principle those same ideals of autonomous human persons in progressive societies. These are societies in which a wide range of human rights are acknowledged and respected and in which institutions are available to provide for democratic or democratically inspired adjustment to new social realities.[1] Thus we have reasons both ideal and factual in support of our free choice of these ideals. While this is not a definitively compelling argument for these ideals and these alone, if the general scheme of reality here is correct, it may be the best argument available. Reason on our account does not stand outside

26

events and it cannot provide "proofs" for matters concerning the relationship of ideal and fact. Instead, reason operates within real contexts and it seizes on considerations which can make a free choice in that context a responsible one. From the practical standpoint, the ultimate argument for this choice is its usefulness in concrete medical contexts. This remains to be shown. For now, let us accept as initially plausible the choice of the ideals of autonomous human persons in progressive societies as ideals ideally and factually worth considering in greater detail and worth applying speculatively to the contemporary medical context.

The ideal of an autonomous human person, as we have seen, is the ideal of a person freely and rationally transcending himself or herself by the progressive creation and application of ideals. It must be possible then for that aspect of the total human person which we call the self to make free and rational choices. The total human person, of course, includes the body and other public facts, but we will now ignore these facts for the sake of exploring the ongoing choice making ability of the most intimately private aspect of the person, the self. It must also be possible for this ongoing process of the self to be a genuine ideal, that is, something we can take to be admirable in itself. This view of the self will then be the core of our ideal of the autonomous person. To show this, certain key dimensions of the human self will have to be explored.[2]

During the greater part of my day, I live in a public world. I met and speak with other persons; I engage with them in activities of work and play; I live with them and outside of myself. Nevertheless, there is an aspect of my life as a whole person which is intrinsically private. I have, for example, my own experiences of pleasures and pains. Though it is usually very easy to know when another person is in pleasure or in pain by a smile, a frown, or any part of the whole range of behaviors we immediately associate with the feelings of pleasure and pain, we all know of cases when we have felt pleasure or pain and have disguised these feelings in our behavior. Also, we all know of cases in which we suspect that other persons have done this as well. Consider the pleasure we sometimes feel but disguise when some obnoxious individual is embarrassed in front of us by an unknowing third party. Or consider the various pains of headache, indigestion, or boredom which are routinely disguised for the sake of conducting ourselves with others. This human ability, my human ability, to literally feel one thing and display another is evidence of the privacy of the self, of my self. It is a concrete experience of the distinction between the public and the private. No one else feels my pleasures, my pains.

I can also speak to myself. Though it is quite plain that my speech was learned from others in what is nearly a paradigmatic case of socialization, once my language was acquired, it became possible for me to engage myself with inner speech. This is primarily how I think when I am alone: I recall, I anticipate, I consider to myself in internal speech. Such inner speech is graphic when it precedes some of life's fundamental decisions, as in the long private talks designed to sort out possibilities and clarify

27

reasons for choices related to career, marriage, important relations with others, etc. But it is also evident in the short daily remarks made to the self, remarks like: "I mustn't forget to. . .", What is that person's name?", "How long is this going to last?". All of this speech could be made public just as it could be spoken aloud. The important fact is that it is not. My inner speech is a private mental reserve wherein I freely consider what I do not share with others. No one else thinks my thoughts.

Finally, though I often display them to others in gesture and in speech, my emotions are private as felt. My emotions may well be products of education by others but the experience of them is mine alone. Even when others can see that I am happy, they do not experience my feeling of happiness. Even when others can accurately predict that some event will inevitably exhilarate or depress me, I alone know the giddiness of my exhilaration and the lethargy of my depression. No one else feels my emotions.

In most general terms, though my body and my speech are public facts, my consciousness is private. Though I clearly live with others, I am essentially alone, the center of my own consciousness. You can enter my consciousness and I can enter yours only indirectly and vicariously. My world, therefore, is **the** world. What occurred before I was aware is history and no part of my world of direct experience. What will occur after my death is the imponderable future and no part of my direct experience. The birth and death of my consciousness are the lived limits of the world for me. And because the dawn of my consciousness is shrouded in the mist of early half-memories, the primary personal fact of my world is the inevitability of its termination. I will die a personal death which no one can die with me or for me. The privacy and individuality of my death is a symbol for the privacy and individuality of my life, my world, my self.[3]

It is this privacy that makes me capable of being radically free. I feel pleasure or pain but I choose whether and how to display it. I conduct a lengthy private reasoning but freely choose if it is to be revealed, to whom, and to what extent. I feel a whole range of emotions but chose whether or not to convey them, to act them out. I know that my life is my own life and my death will be my own death. This personal knowing places all my life's choices in a new and radical framework: If I do anything with this unique and limited world of experience, I do so as a free use of a rare and diminishing resource. The inevitability of my death and the brevity of my life before it adds drama and urgency to my ability to choose freely. Against this background, the press of events and the demands of others are as nothing if I choose not to have them in my world. As no one else dies my death, so no one else can command my free choices in life.

But the knowledge of my freedom has a consequence. Freedom entails responsibility.[4] If I am free to choose, then I am responsible for what I choose, have chosen, and will choose. After so radicalizing my world, it is no option to say that he or she made me do something, or that everyone expected that I would do something, or even that I allowed pure caprice to dictate my doing something. My choices, even where they have clear social dimensions as when others place demands on me; my choices are mine and I alone am ultimately responsible for them. Just as the public character of life often disguises my private death and private freedom within the nonreflective unity of ordinary consciousness, so it also tends to disguise my ultimate responsibility. Nevertheless, it is clear on reflection that each of my actions is a voluntary use of my limited consciousness before death for which I alone can be held responsible. The weight of this responsibility, if seriously shouldered, will bring a being capable of it to reasoning. Since I am free and thus responsible, I want to use my freedom to the best possible advantage, a best possible advantage I can only identify for myself if I am willing and able to clarify, organize, and criticize my experience. Thus my freedom and responsibility drives me to reason. This point does not exclude acknowledgement of the emotive and habit-based character of most of my choices. Generally I do what is satisfying or what I usually do or both. But if I am to use this precious resource of my world wisely, I must periodically reason to educate my emotions and to inspect and redirect my habits. Thus the privacy of my consciousness, the very nature of my self and its apparent limitation leads me to the desire to use my freedom and reason to their fullest.

This self that I live with and freely and reasonably expend is also the source of all value in my world. It is obvious but revealing to note that no person, place, activity has value in itself unless it has value for me. Of course, from a social perspective, there are many values I am unaware of — persons, places, and activities taken as valuable by knowledgeable others. Yet if they make up no part of my world they make up no part of **the** world since my world is **the** world for me. Unless I bring a value to my self in some fashion, unless I invest it with my self, it is no value for me in my world. Only if I decide that this person is worth the use of a portion of my life, does he or she become a value for me. Only if I decide that this place is worth the use of my limited attention does it become a value for me. Only if I decide that this activity is worth the use of my exhaustible energies does it become a value for me. Obviously, most values do not enter our lives in such a reflective fashion but through spontaneous feelings and habitual actions. That this is not actually the way values enter into our lives is beside the point at hand. Logically, the source of all value is my free commitment of my self. It is the risk of a portion of this fragile and transitory self that brings a value into my world. Even if my embrace of a value is wholly unreflective, it is still this devoting of my passing self to persons, things, and activities beyond it that gives these experiences value.[5]

The self, then, is the source of all of life's values and is, therefore, itself the value of values. It is the ultimate cause of what I most truly want, of what I most truly do, of what I most truly am. The having of any other values thus implies a tacit valuing of the self. By contrast, to deny the self value would be to remove all value from the world. It is hard to imagine that I could continue to value anything else in my experience if there was not this implicit valuing of my self. Were I to consciously regard my self as valueless, how could I value other persons, things, activities? These would all pass by me as meaningless, as meaningless as our value worlds likely appear to nonself-conscious animals. But to value these persons, things, and activities is to value them for my self and through my self. This notion of the self as the free and (potentially) reasonable source of all values therefore makes my self the value of my world. Because this is so, the possibility that this self can continue to freely and reasonably create and articulate other values strikes me as a conceived state of affairs admirable in itself, that is, it strikes me with the force of an ideal. The inherent attractiveness of the possibility of a continuously free and rational self transcending itself through the creation of values is the meaning of the ideal of the human person as autonomous. My autonomy as a complete person just is my ability to freely and reasonably confer value on persons, things, and activities through the process of drawing these things into my world, bringing them to that aspect of my person that is my self. The protection and enhancement of personal autonomy therefore appears a reasonable choice of an ideal to freely embrace.

This is not to say that autonomy entails selfishness. Selfishness is the fault of developing a habit of too great a concern for what is in one's narrow self-interest, too great a concern for one's own share of pleasure, money, fame, etc. Selfishness is properly condemned both because it is prejudicial against the interests of others and because it distracts the self from its true self-interest most broadly construed. Acts of self-sacrifice, charity, and concern for others in general are not only socially useful and protective of the interests of others, but they are also ennobling and expansive of the self. An act of charity, for example, opens the self to interpersonal awareness and personal growth in a manner which an act of selfishness can not. Thus emphasis on the role of the self in the construction of the ideal of autonomous persons is not selfishness; instead it is the necessary emphasis for understanding how any value can become a value. Since these values can and should include other directed values in a most genuine fashion, the development of autonomous persons, of free and rational value creating selves, is the precondition for all values whether self directed or other directed. All other values rely on a prior and implicit valuing of the self.[6]

B. The Self and Society

The self as just described, the self which is free, rational, and the source of all values, is an ideal elaborated from that aspect of our experience which is private. But the self, like all realities, is not only ideal, but is also bound to the fact world. In fact, the private self is only an aspect of the whole person, a person with a body, and public emotions, habits, and social relationships. These facts can facilitate or frustrate the realization of the ideal of personal autonomy, as they make for or work against the real development of practical autonomy. A person whose body is so racked with pain or so compromised by dysfunction that concern for the body dominates all experience can hardly be practically free. A person whose mind is so beset by untamed passions or inappropriate emotions can hardly be practically rational. A person whose experience is so private as to be estranged from society will hardly have values that can be practically respected and reinforced by others. Recognition of these facts is incumbent on those who would make their ideals more real. Let us consider some of the more significant facts that relate to our ideal of personal autonomy and which facilitate or frustrate its practical attainment.

The body in general is a social inheritance as we have seen, our DNA representing generations of the passing on of our species' genetic and environmental interactions. The body in particular is the concrete vehicle of the person. Sickness or serious impairment of the body can dramatically reduce the chances for attaining practical autonomy. Medical care, improved santitation and nutrition, and greater public awareness of the causes of sickness and wellness in our environment have dramatically improved the character of the average human bodily experience in terms both of an increase in the number of days of adequate functioning and freedom from pain and in terms of the extension of the span of the average human life. Still, short of the completion of medical advance in all of its variety, one must acknowledge a tremendous element of luck in our lives and in our real abilities to become autonomous. To be born free of deleterious genetic mutation, to have access to proper sanitation and nutrition, and to escape the sundry physical risks associated with human life is no less than good fortune. Any factually relevant ideal of human autonomy must recognize this element of chance in life. Many human persons are born with or happen into such disabilities that personal autonomy is not a meaningful goal. Embracing the ideal of personal autonomy against this background of chance implies an obligation to try to minimize the many harms of bad luck. It implies an obligation to advance medical care and to pacify the many physical hazards of our environment so as to maximize the percentage of human persons reasonably capable of seeking to realize a practical measure of personal autonomy in their lives.

We have already admitted the great role of emotions and habits in our lives. These pervasive dimensions of experience are largely shaped by our culture, the random facts of our lives, and by conscious choice. However the emotions and habits of any given person are formed, they will have a considerable impact on the possibility of attaining meaningful personal autonomy. Cultures, situations, and choices which lead to radically inappropriate emotions or to hidebound habits can diminish or even extinguish practical personal autonomy. Embracing the ideal of personal autonomy here implies an obligation to critique and change such factors as well.

Perhaps the single most important aspect of our individual lives which makes for or inhibits the realization of practical personal autonomy is our social world and its many expressions.[7] The privacy of our consciousness is but one pole of our lives; the other is the totality of our public relationships. The character of the society within which we grow and live shapes our concrete horizons as individual persons. Society fashions our interpretations of the past and our expectations for the future. It summarizes in its institutions the achievements persons have already attained and sets the stage in these same institutions for the possibility of further achievements. The nature and structure of these social institutions, therefore, have a profound effect on the ability of any single person in society to secure meaningful personal autonomy.

The clearest example of this intrinsically social nature of the human person and one of its first expressions is the language acquisition of the child. Beginning from genetically determined behaviors like sucking, crying, and babbling the child begins to imitate the speech of other persons the social world. The rambling baby talk of the small child gradually conforms to the meaningful linguistic structures of the adult world. The child learns to substitute words for pointing and ideas for experiences and thus comes to convey complex thoughts and feelings through the conventions of language. There is a powerful socialization implied here. To learn a language is to enter a world. Study of foreign languages suggests that each tongue not only makes the world intelligible to its speakers, but that it also does so in a slightly idiosyncratic fashion. The language of the English speaking world brings one's attention to slightly different phenomena and to the same phenomena in a slightly different fashion than the language of the French speaking or Chinese speaking worlds. This is so because every natural language describes the world in terms of the emotions and habits of its speakers. Language is a way of structuring a world, and each language does so in a way unique to its own history and present reality. Thus language acquisition is at once the acquisition of a social world.[8] Both of these self-defining acquisitions come to us before we are capable of autonomous choice. Indeed, a language and a social world are key prior ingredients for the real development of personal autonomy.

Furthermore, the acquisition of language is the acquisition, for all practical purposes, of the skill of reasoning. There may indeed be reasonings without words, but if there are they are far overwhelmed in number by the great bulk of our reasonings which are verbal whether spoken aloud or privately to oneself. Reasoning depends on language and is thus a social skill. One learns to reason by hearing and reading the reasonings of others. Reasoning, as has already been pointed out, also has a private use as inner speech. But inner speech is quite likely an achievement which is possible only after one has learned outer speech, just as learning to read to oneself is generally preceded by learning to read aloud to others. Inner speech like inner reading depends first on an external learning from others in society. Consequently, my very ability to define and enrich my self through the medium of inner speech is an ability owed to the society of those around me. My would-be rational self is thus a social achievement. And since reason is central to my autonomy, this too is a social achievement in part.

The imitations of the very young in language acquisition and in the learning of a multitude of other human skills is mirrored throughout the rest of an individual's life in countless ways. In adolescence, for example, just when one might expect to see signs of the maturation of personal autonomy, there appears the most compelling urge to conform to one's peers. Such teenage conformism asserts itself in our society even in the midst of the glorification of individualism and even as whole aspects of the adult world are being criticized and rejected. This drive to be accepted is a psychologically powerful expression of our social nature. We want the people that matter to us to think well of us; we want our autonomous choices confirmed by significant others in our society. Though this specific phenomenon is strongly associated with adolescence, it is not unlike the social urge that runs throughout the adult world. Consciously or not, we seem always and everywhere to seek the approval of those who matter most to us, of spouses, parents, children, friends, coworkers, neighbors, etc. These approvals or disapprovals from the society around us are powerful forces for the facilitation or frustration of practical autonomy.

Even in the most ideal cases, that of the practically autonomous adult, there is still the ineluctable social dimension of the search for life's meaning. Few adults, even the most autonomous, will be satisfied with the idea that the meaning of life is wholly private, is wholly what I or you or he or she makes of it. For most people, this is roughly equivalent to saying that life itself has no meaning. Thus a totally private meaning appears as no meaning at all. Acceptable answers must be more public; they must say that "everyone's life is meaningful because. . ." or "the nature of all life is such that. . ." or that "inevitably all of us. . ." There is no avoiding the clear social urge here. One finds meaning personally when that meaningfulness is thought to be there for all of us socially. We seem to have an intuitive sense that for beings so similar in so many ways, there must be some single answer, some stable public meaning for life. Perhaps this sense is only the felt anxiety of a self which finds that it must choose freely for itself and therefore looks to others for security. Perhaps this sense points to something more significant about the shared character of our search for meaning. In any event, the sense that life's meaning must be publicly there for all of us is powerful evidence of our social nature. And the meaning we finally find in life can graphically affect the possibility of attaining practical personal autonomy.

These examples of the many social dimensions of the human person suggest the idea of viewing the self as a concrete microcosm of society. The individual self on this account can be conceived of as a small society itself.[9] Just as society is a complex of institutions, social roles, and multiple communities of persons with interests, so the individual self can be conceived as a complex of habits, social roles, and multiple communities of interests within the self. As the institutions of a society set in motion routine feelings and actions, so habits do the same for each person. Social roles are played out on large scale as in the cases of holders of national offices, leading figures in commerce and the arts, representatives of large communities and groups, etc, but they are also played out in small interpersonal intimacies as in the cases of spouses, parents, children, friends, etc. These intimate roles determine and shape the self. In many respects, a person just is the concrete intersection of all of his or her various social roles, public as well as intimate. Communities of special interests and goals abound within society at large, but, in a sense, they also abound within the self. The business concern, labor union, or organized church are like larger expressions of dimensions of myself, of the interests within me that seek financial stability, fair working conditions, and access to religious worship. The individual self can even be regarded as a society of differing selves related and overlapping in time. As there are multiple relationships between persons in a society, so there are multiple relationships between the self I was as a child, the self I am now, and the self I anticipate I will be in the future.

This point may fairly be reversed as well. If the self can be conceived to be a concrete microcosm of society, society can be thought of as an abstract macrocosm of the self. Societies display public emotions in their ceremonies and rituals and fixed habits of action in their institutions. Societies have public values related to their collective perceptions of facts and of ideals, perceptions exhibited in the many activities of curiosity and creativity pervading a society. Societies can, through political and cultural mechanisms, make free and reasonable choices. Furthermore, there is something like a public mind in a society, a phenomenon clearly visible when a society faces some great event such as war, novel technology, or economic change. At times like these, a whole society can feel, think, and act with a unity approaching that typical of an individual self.

Given this analogy between the character of the self and society and given the fact that society sets the horizon for the facts and ideals with which persons concretely realize or fail to realize the ideal of autonomy; given these assumptions, it is critical that society and social change be brought under the control of an ideal consistent with the ideal of personal autonomy. The ideal of personal autonomy is equivalent to the ideal of a self continually transcending himself or herself through free and rational choice. The analogous ideal in society then would be that of a society which continually transcends itself through free and rational choice at the public level. Such a society would be able to continually adjust and improve the conditions under which persons in that society express their own practical autonomy in the face of changing facts and ideals. In short, it would be a progressive society.

Since society is no real self at all, but only analogously so, the actual free and rational choices of society will of necessity be those of real persons. Therefore, a society can approach the goal of being a progressive society only if it structures its main institutions, especially but not exclusively its political ones, in ways which allow for the free participation of autonomous persons at all levels of social life. This means that democratic political and social institutions will be defining characteristics of a pro-

34

gressive society.[10] Democratic social habits maximize free participation of autonomous persons throughout society and thus assure the widest range of freedom and reason in social choices. Just as inappropriately strong emotions and inflexible habits can make the realization of autonomy factually impossible in a person, so extreme traditionalism and authoritarian political and social institutions can make the realization of autonomy factually impossible in a society as a whole. Practical personal autonomy and democratic social autonomy thus reinforce one another. The making of large numbers of autonomous persons requires a progressive society; the creation of a progressive society requires the commitment of large numbers of autonomous persons. Both ideals can be approached only if there is an increasing amount of active, free, and reasonable participation by persons in all of the social aspects of their lives. Thus our ideal of the autonomous person implies a companion ideal of a progressive society — a society which can freely and rationally transcend itself to more fully realize its collective ideals and can thus set increasingly favorable factual and ideal conditions for the making of autonomous persons.

C. Dignity and Human Rights

Self, society, and their participatory interaction constitute the framework for the structure of the ideals of personal and social autonomy. Both therefore express themselves in our moral experience as concrete values. An experience of the concrete value of the self is available to each self on reflection, as has been shown. The value of society follows from the fact that it is composed of persons, themselves capable of such a reflective experience of self value. Society embodies in its practices the emotions, habits, and free choices of persons of the past. These institutional emotions, habits, and free choices compose the starting point for the formation of the autonomous persons of tomorrow. For these reasons and for the countless other goods of society — friendships, productive work and stimulating play, the riches of culture, etc. — society is a value.

But the value of society must be conceived to be second in worth to that of the human person. The value that I find at the heart of my private self is the value of all values since it is the creator of values in my world. This makes the value of myself incalculably great, that is, quite beyond any numerical appraisal or fixing of any sort. Drawn out abstractly this way, my value as a self appears to me as absolute. It is outside market mechanisms for determining relative value. To conceive of the self in this fashion is to recognize its essential dignity, its incalculable worth. The dignity of the self thus establishes a permanent gulf between the world of persons and the world of things.[11] Each thing, regardless of how precious it may be, has a price; a relative value determinable by the thing's relationship to other goods or services, its relative scarcity, and the strength of persons' desires for it. But my person as the valuing and valued self it is, is beyond all pricing because its value is incalculable and absolute. My self, therefore, has a dignity which animates my entire being as a human person.

35

At the same time, I know that my ability to have this dignity concretely and to realize the ideal of an autonomous person ever more fully is very much a function of the society I am within. There can be social situations in which a person is so degraded by reduction to a price equivalence that little meaningful content is left for the claims of dignity. Slavery, for example, is the abomination that it is because it is a straightforward assault on personal dignity. The slave is made into a thing by being made directly equivalent to a relative price. And there are other more subtle forms of slavery of the person, of reduction of a person to a thing, carried on even in the most progressive of contemporary societies: physical and mental prostitutions, meaningless and mind killing labor, relationships in which one party trades personal dignity for security, fame, or pleasure. Thus the dignity of the self as the core of the ideal of personal autonomy is also a social accomplishment, or failure, in fact. Consequently, my concern for the preservation of my dignity cannot simply be a private and ideal one. Instead, it must also assert itself in the public world of fact as the demand for criticism and change of all social habits which assault human dignity.

Futhermore, it is clear that society is not only its institutions and practices but more fundamentally it is a world of other persons. It is true that I have no direct access to the private selves of other persons, and thus I cannot experience the value creation of their worlds. Nevertheless, the concrete selves of other persons are shown factually in what these persons say and do. Excepting the direct access I have to my own inner world, what other persons say and do appears remarkably similar to what I say and do. I note others valuing persons, places, and activities. Some of these values are my own values too. I note the emotions, habits, and choices of others. Sometimes I almost share these same emotions as when the crying of another brings me to tears or when the laughter of another turns my world comic and laughable. The habits of others are remarkably like my own from the automatic body gestures of stress or relaxation to the highly choice controlled habits of driving an automobile, exchanging small talk, and balancing moments of society and privacy. The choices of others often appear to be free and rational, and they can and do have real effects on me. Sometimes I reason with other persons and as I do I see, for all the differences and debates, a skill at work remarkably similar to my own.

Futhermore, I know as a matter of fact that these similarities are not happenstance. I know others have emotions and habits like mine since I know we share, many of us, a common cultural inheritance. I know others choose freely and reasonably as I do since I can remember being taught this skill by others and I have myself shared in its teaching. In short, I have very good reasons to think that the selves of other persons are remarkably similar to my own even though I do not experiences theirs' directly as I do mine. It is the most reasonable of guesses, in fact an unconscious presumption of all social life, that all other persons are selves who on reflection can take themselves to be absolute values.

36

This insight suggests that dignity is not my private possession but a social accomplishment ture, at least in ideal, of all and every human person. Thus, every persons in ideal has the dignity of an incalculably worthy value of values. This, in turn, means that all persons are similarly distanced from the world of things. No human person should ever be priced or made equivalent to any other value. Neither can persons be interchaned as things are. Though the value of each person is absolute and thus equal, the absolute value of each individual person follows from the unique and private vantage point of each value creating self. This is the ultimate individuality that remains for persons even when we have admitted their vast similarity and even when we have admitted that all absolute values are equal in ideal. Persons are radically different because of the privacy of their value creative activity, but radically equal in the absolute value attributable to each person because of that value creative activity.

Contemporary human societies, especially those sharing the cultural assumptions of the western democracies, have begun to recognize this dignity of each human person. Though this advance is not the exclusive property of these societies, the very fact of their democratice, thus progressive, political institutions serves to insure and accelerate this result. In the facts of their organized religions, their legal systems, their social conventions, and in the emotions and habits of the individual persons produced by these societies, the political democracies are creating favorable factual conditions for the making of large numbers of autonomous persons. In these societies the dominant Judeo-Christian religious tradition preaches the dignity of the individual person as the creation of a personal God.[12] The Anglo-American and Roman legal systems defend the dignity of persons in their civil relationships and when accused of crime.[13] The social conventions of these democracies, of civility, aid to the needy, and support for free individual human achievement in all of its variety express this same value.[14] These societies are providing the cultural horizons against which more and more individual persons are developing their own practical autonomy and with it a spontaneous and habitual "feel" for the dignity of all persons. If the scheme presented above is accurate then the making of such large numbers of increasinlgy autonomous persons will bring with it more pressure for the further democratization of these nations' social habits. Thus these societies are in a position to factually transcend themselves.

This is not social naivete, blind to darker realities. Everywhere, even in these democracies, there are assults on human dignity and the existence of social practices which make the concrete expression of dignity impossible. The twentieth century has seen some of the worst cruelties and inhumanities ever inflicted by persons on one another. The political democracies of the West are not without substantial responsibility for these cruelties and inhumanities. Furthermore, even in the most ideally progressive society, there will always be the inevitable distance between ideal and fact, between what ought to be and what is. Nevertheless, it appears to be a growing social fact that vigorous commitment to the ideals of autonomous persons in progressive societies, and to the protection of human dignity which these ideals entail, is having a factual effect on these society.[15] As it does, we are being placed in a better position to further clarify, organize, and critique these ideals, to commit ourselves to further realize them in fact and thus to continue the process of transcendence already described. At the very least, political democracies open themsleves institutionally to the possibility of such improvement and thus allow for a reasonable hope.

This discussion of dignity leads to another notion central to the ideal of personal autonomy and one closely associated with accomplishments in the realization of that ideal in progressive societies: human rights. The having of dignity gives rise to the having of rights. If the human person has the dignity we have described, then the human person ought not to have that dignity assaulted. Persons ought to have the ability to make claims for dignity on other persons and on their socieites in general. Such claims for dignity are assertions of fundamental rights. The rights of persons are thus instrumental expressions of their dignities. Persons have rights because as incalcuably great values there are things it would be wrong to do to them. First among these wrongs are actions which directly assault the possibility of achieving human dignity; actions like murder, slavery, and torture. These actions deny to persons the status of an incalculably great value. The first and rudimentary right of all persons, then, is the right to be accorded that status of a person, the status of being a self with dignity.

As instrumental expressions of the ideal dignity, rights may be thought of as one step closer to the fact world. Internal to rights themselves, we can distinguish between those that have worked themselves largely into fact already, as in the case of legal rights, and those whose status remains more ideal but whose assertion still makes for a factually relevant appeal to members of a given society, as in the case of claims for moral rights not codified into law. If the account of reality given here is adequate, we should exprect to see a continuing movement of moral rights into legal rights as the ideal world becomes me factually realized. The claims, therefore, of moral rights are far from being empty and useless simply because they are not legally recognized. Such claims are the absolutely necessary precondition for such rights becoming legal fact. Calims for moral rights begin the process of clarification, organization, and critque of our dieal and factual worlds and set the stage for new moral realities. It is fact, for example, that the moral assertions of the Declaration of Independence preceded the legal structure of the U.S. Consitution, and that the ideal claims of abolitionists preceded the factual termination of American slavery. It will likely be the fact that many of the moral rights in today's manifestos will be the accomplished legal facts of the future.[16]

Since rights move dignity into closer connection with the world of fact, the determination of what are the rights of human persons will require not only consideration of our ideals but also close attention to fact. The facts are that human dignity can be made impossible in the concrete either by the active oppression of society or other persons, or by lack of access to those goods and services known to be necessary for a life of human dignity. Thus we recognize negative rights or rights of personal liberty, such as rights to be free of others' interference with life, movement, thought, associations, relationship to God, etc. And we recognize positive rights or rights of access to the factual necessities of a life with human dignity, such as rights to adequate nutrition, housing, health care, education, productive labor, and old age security.[17]

All of these rights are imperfectly realized even in the progressive societies that have acknowledged and codified them into law and some societies, even among the most progressive, still refuse to acknowledge some of these rights. The recognition of and respect for a full range of individual rights, both negative and positive, is a clear mark of a truly progressive society. Social autonomy requires the fullest possible participation of all autonomous persons and that in turn can only begin to be possible when human dignity is protected and enhanced by respect for the rights of individual persons. There seems to be a growing human consensus that a life of dignity, a life fit for an autonomous human person, can be made possible only if certain negative and positive rights are admitted in ideal as mal rights and brought into fact as legal rights. Whatever the factual variability of these rights, positive and negative, moral and legal, there is one final point about rights that follows from our ideal of the human person. As all humans beings are possessed of dignity, so human rights are universla in ideal. All and every human person has the same human rights. This is the concrete expression of our ideals of autonomous persons in progressive societies.

II. Tools to Realize the Ideal: Morality and Ethics

Chapter 4.

Morality

A. Intuitions of Value and of Duty

There are many kinds of ideals. For example, there are ideals of method, those ideals of objectivity, consistency, and accuracy which constitute the core of scientific inquiry and of logic and mathematics. There are also aesthetic ideals of how life is to be lived with grace and beauty. There are religious ideals as to how a person should stand before God and of holiness and saintly behavior. There are military ideals, ideals of productive labor, ideals of fulfilling leisure, ideals of family life and of living alone, etc. It is hard to be very precise when dealing with ideals not only because they are as pervasive as human reality itself, but also because they are inherently vague. This is not a problem of our inability to know ideals fully. Rather ideals, because of their necessary remove from fact, are not in themselves fully determined. Even those who espouse verbally the same ideal can differ dramatically on the implications that ideal has for practice. This does not mean that someone is necessarily wrong or disingenuous here. Ideals open themselves to various interpretations by their very indeterminate being. This openness of ideals can become gradually concretized by the events of history. For example, it likely would have shocked most signers of the Declaration of Independence in the 18th century to assert that the ideal of all men being created equal entails racial equality. This implication was drawn out more clearly by 19th century abolitionists and made relatively concrete by the emotions and habits produced by the 20th century civil rights movement.

One way of grasping the character of an ideal more fully is to look at which values it generates in the concrete. A value is something which shares the intrinsically attractive nature of an ideal but does so in a more specific and factually relevant fashion. An ideal motivates my action in general; a value moves me in particular circumstances. If I embrace the ideal of autonomous persons, then I will likely value activities which make persons more free and rational, activities such as education, free exchange of information and ideas, and respect for persons' rights. Values can become very specific and very concrete such as in the specific desire to learn this fact, the exchange of this idea, the respect for this right. An ideal

40

is what we might admit motivates us overall and in the long run when we reflect about it; a value is what we show as our motivation here and now and with little or no reflection.

The ideals that most concern us here, the autonomy of persons in progressive societies, could, if developed in different fashions, be thought of as aesthetic, religious, or even methodological ideals but they are primarily moral ideals, i.e., ideals having to do with how we ought to act towards ourselves and towards one another in society. When ideals animate and regulate a society's morality, the spontaneous moral responses of members of that society will be to grasp for the values which are concretely derivative from those ideals. A better understanding of the nature of morality, then, should help to clarify the ideals we have chosen here and should improve our ability to use this tool on behalf of those ideals. Central to a better understanding of morality is an examination of valuing.

Let us call the specific act of the valuing of a concrete something in the here and now, an intuition. This word captures the fact that at the lived level, a specific value is grasped for immediately and without reflection.[1] An intuition of value is a spontaneously felt "knowing" that this is the object or activity I want now. From the spontaneously felt "knowing" that I want more cream in my coffee to the spontaneously felt "knowing" that this person needs my active assistance right now, our lives are replete with value intuitions. To develop a sense for the ubiquity of valuing, simply consider the many persons, objects, and activities that attract our attention and efforts each day. It would be more than hard to conceive of a human person or human society in which value intuitions were not this all-pervasive.

The value intuitions most specific to morality are those couched in terms of good and bad. It is a matter of fact that our moralities provide us with value intuitions that this is good and that is bad, for example, that this act of kindness is good and that act of cruelty is bad. Similarly, we judge as good or bad persons and their characteristics, natural and artificial objects of all sorts, animals and their actions, and the whole panoply of human activities. There is hardly an experience which could not be and is not judged by some persons to be good or bad. Morality also displays another major category of intuitions, viz., those of duty, of right and wrong. As moral persons, we have duty intuitions that this act needs to be done and that that act must be refrained from, for example, that this promise must be fulfilled just now and that I must refrain now from articulating the insult I feel welling up inside me. There is a wide range of similar duty intuitions though perhaps not as wide as those of value. While we may feel duties to some animals and things, for example, a felt duty to preserve the quality of our natural environment, intuitions of duty arise primarily with respect to persons. There is a complex and delicate relationship between value and duty, between intuitions of good and bad and intuitions of right and wrong. It is clearly a human value, for instance, that persons do their duty. It is also clear that duty itself would be purely formal and mean-

41

ingless unless it were related somehow to our values. Perhaps a tentative suggestion of this relationship is all that is needed here since this point will be explored more fully as we proceed. It appears that values, because of their intrinsic attractiveness and their relationship to more general ideals, are progressive and dynamic: They lead us to grasp for and seek to enjoy a wider range of moral satisfactions. Duties, on the other hand, appear inhibitory and conservative: They demand that we preserve the achievements of our moral past even as we grasp for more in the future. For instance, I may have a chance to secure a significant value for myself; I am powerfully drawn to it. But suppose that I have promised someone else something incompatible with my securing this value just now; I feel a powerful duty which inhibits my drive to secure this value. Thus values appear to comprise the drive and content of moral advance as duties comprise the stability and structure of moral accomplishment. Even as my values drive me to seek to expand my practical personal autonomy, for example, I "know" intuitively that I have a duty not to do so at another person's expense. Even as we feel collectively that we ought to seek to enhance the possibilities for attainment of values for all, we also feel a duty to do so without violating the rights of persons so far achieved. Some of life's most difficult moral problems arise out of this interaction of value and duty, out of this clash between deeply felt attractions and inhibitions.

In order to clarify these points further, it is necessary to distinguish between morality and ethics. It is common for persons to use the words 'morality' and 'ethics' interchangeably without change in meaning. In spite of this prevailing usage, for the sake of clarity, let us stipulate a distinction. For the purposes at hand, 'morality' will be used to refer to the specific system of intuitions of value and duty prevailing in a society at a given time and to those same intuitions of value and duty as they express themselves in the contextual unity of the lived experience of individual persons. Thus every human person and every society has a morality. Needless to say, what morally attracts one society may be repugnant to another and what one person feels duty bound to do may appear optional or even forbidden to another. In other words, to attribute a morality to all persons and societies is not to say that all persons and societies have values and duties which we would find acceptable as a society or as individual persons. Instead, the attribution of a morality to all persons and societies is an assertion of the fundamentally moral character of all human experience: The person and society with no values and no duties is quite literally inconceivable. We would find more in common with the value of a criminal who seeks stolen goods or a cannibal who feels a duty to eat the heart of his enemy than with beings who found nothing immediately attractive and nothing immediately obligatory. We would not recognize our species in such beings because morality, as defined here, is as clearly a human species characteristic as reason, speech, and the opposable thumb. All human societies have had and do have moralities. By contrast to this use of 'morality,' 'ethics' will be reserved to refer to conscious reflections about morality. Thus morality is what we do naturally and nonreflectively and ethics is the reflective study of this natural and nonreflective knowing and doing.

Our moralities are carried socially in the values and duties structured into our social habits generally but especially in our religious traditions, legal systems, and social conventions, including the received view of proper child rearing. These institutions and the practices combine to produce in the individual human person what we call a conscience, i.e., the earnest and spontaneous having of intuitions of value and duty and the will to act on these intuitions. Thus society provides a conventional structuring of our natural disposition toward having moral intuitions. This action of society is so constant and so subtle in most cases that it results in what appears to most people as a naturally given morality. In many cases, it is only after the shock of encountering radically differing moral intuitions that one realizes the conventional character of much of one's inherited morality. Except when this insight prevails, morality appears to be a second nature because of the spontaneity with which it expresses itself and because of the constant reinforcements of one's moral intuitions by members of one's own society. Those within our own society without the conventional moral intuitions seem wicked, morally blind, or the products of poor moral education. Such persons are criticized, blamed, and in extreme cases, punished. The power of the conventions of morality are so strong that such judgments of other persons and their actions generally appear to be straightforward and obvious, as straightforward and as obvious as the description of a natural state of affairs.

Further, these moral intuitions are forcefully emotional. Our intuitions are as much felt as they are thought and in both cases with strength, immediacy, and a sense of confidence. One need think here only of the context within which a child is taught to be moral, for instance to be truthful or not to hurt another, to see the complex intertwining of emotions and thoughts carried in our moral intuitions.[2] A whole range of rewards and punishments are employed to build the desired emotional associations as well as to regulate the building of habits. Parents deliberately and properly cause their children to feel good emotionally when they have been good morally and to feel bad emotionally when they have been bad morally. This emotional dimension of morality is longstanding and for most people constantly reinforced in future behavior. Even the most highly reflective of individuals often finds himself or herself with strong feelings for a conventional moral intuition long after he or she has consciously rejected the rational grounds for that intuition. Our moralities are an intimate part of our entire emotional lives and vice versa.

That our conventional moralities are spontaneous, nonreflective, and emotion filled is no criticism of them. The function of morality is to regulate and control action, and successful action requires quick, sure, and emotionally satisfying responses to the stimuli of our natural and social environment. The morally mature person has an intuitive and finely tuned sense of good and bad, right and wrong, and this sense is the guide for his or her actions. Such a person is a satisfied individual, a consummate social achievement, and the stuff of which great cultures are made.

B. The Morally Unique and the Morally Similar

There is a respect in which the exercise of each moral intuition by each person in each situation is a radically unique event.[3] If the total moral situation is composed of the relevant moral intuition, the person as agent, and the set of circumstances within which the moral intuition occurs, then no two moral situations are ever wholly alike. The person as agent has as an aspect a unique self, a self differing in some respect from all other selves. Even in the case of identical twins raised by the same parents, each twin will have some experiences which differ from the other and thus will be a different and unique self. Even a repeated intuition by the same agent differs from the first instance of the intuition by virtue of the fact that the agent now brings the first intuition as a latent memory to the situation of the second. If the self is comprised in part of its own history of experiences and the latent memories which result from them, then no two temporal selves of the same person are ever truly the same regardless of how close they may be to one another. And, of course, most of us are just plainly different selves from those around us.

Also the general circumstances of the intuition will vary. Most putatively similar intuitions of value or duty will occur in spatially different locations and our equally intuitive sense of place will affect the character of these intuitions. A felt duty to help someone at home will be different on its face from the "same" felt duty at work. In those cases where place is constant, surely time will vary. If time in general is a measure of the changing circumstances of personal and social history, then the very temporal order of two of the "same" intuitions will make them different. Yesterday's felt duty to help someone has become history and that history has an impact on the intuitions of duty to help someone today.

All of these points, valid as they may be, amount to little when compared to the constantly altering specific circumstances within which our intuitions occur. The person at home I feel a duty to help may be a loved one, a spouse, a parent, or a child, while the person I feel a duty to help at work may be a total stranger or even someone I actively dislike. Intuitions of the value of honesty will take vastly differing shapes in the context of work than they will in the context of play, as in the difference between honesty in a legal contract and in a game of poker. The variables which can intervene to radically change or slightly color one circumstance from another are too numerous to name and too obvious to require naming. For all of these reasons, each moral intuition is a unique occurence.

On the other hand, it is clear that we group individual moral intuitions together in classes by naming them. Common names suggest common features. The duty I felt to help someone I love at home yesterday must share some important features with my felt duty to help someone I dislike at work today or we would not call them both cases of duties to help. Naming is a way of categorizing, and categorizing, when reasonable, is a sorting of things into classes on the basis of some similarity. Our world would be pure chaos if names were distributed without such a basis in similarity. Think only of the confusion a child or a foreigner learning English feels in the face of a homonym and this point is clear. Without a basis in similarity for most of our namings, the world would appear through language as a random collection of words that look alike, sound alike, but share no common core of meaning.[4]

Furthermore, if moral intuitions are so radically unique, how is it that we often feel quite confident in our judgments of the adequacy or inadequacy of another person's intuitions? For that matter, how could I, with the self I am now, fairly judge the intuitions of the self I was yesterday? Yet this criticism of others and of oneself, unfair as it may be on occasions, is one of the most palpable facts of all moralities. Moral criticism is a daily occurrence; we judge others and our own past moral intuitions against our present standards. The use of such standards suggests the existence of common features to differing moral intuitions, since without the existence of some common features in our moral intuitions, standards of any sort would be impossible. The only comment one could make of another's moral intuitions or of one's own would be to say that he or she or I had the moral intuitions which, in fact, were had in the circumstances that, in fact, did prevail. No criticism and no standards, and thus no progress in approximating them, could be possible if this were the case. In addition, the asking for and the giving (at times without an asking) of moral advice would be impossible without common features in our moral intuitions. But again, this is too obvious a fact about morality for our intuitions to be so wholly unique.

Perhaps the easiest way to see that our moral intuitions must have some common characteristics in spite of the changing natures of self and circumstances, is to observe that they are learned and taught. One cannot teach what is truly unique to one's own experience nor learn of what is truly unique about another's. The fact of the moral education of the young and the fact of the possibility of the continued moral self-education of the adult belie the claims for the total uniqueness of each moral intuition.

A strategy for reconciling these perspectives of the extreme uniqueness and yet socially accessible character of our moral intuitions is suggested by considering the process through which these intuitions are learned. A young child is taught to judge an object or activity as good, for example, in much the same way he or she is taught the proper usage of any word. Paradigm cases of the object or activity are presented, the word for it pronounced, and the process repeated until the child associates word and experience. 'Good', 'bad', 'right', and 'wrong' are the rudimentary words of moral discourse. These words are learned early, perhaps as early as color words, food words, and family names, and they are learned in this ostensive fashion. As in the case of all word learning, the child is constantly corrected to dispel false associations and is constantly encouraged to notice the nuances of proper usage. It goes without saying that the appropriate emotive resonances are learned together with the learning of the moral

45

words. A smile with the word 'good,' a frown with 'bad' may be all the hints a child needs to begin to feel the appropriate feelings in the face of the word. At a later stage, the child is told stories with patently moral content, learns elementary moral rules, and begins to enter into the shared moral world of the parent and family — the world in which an aunt is good but the dog next door is bad, in which sharing your candy is right but taking someone else's is wrong, etc. One hardly needs the theories of contemporary psychology to see that these early moral intuitions are formative and leave their impress long into adult life.

A point to be observed in this process of learning moral words and in any process of language acquisition is the role of example. The child cannot possibly be taught each and every conceivable use of a moral term, so that this use being taught now is meant to represent, to stand for, an indefinite many other such uses. The story which teaches honesty in this particular case is meant to teach of honesty in general. The rule of not interrupting the speech of another is illustrated by this case of interruption but meant to apply to all others like it. The judgment that this aunt is good inevitably becomes a model for the judging of other relatives, of women, and of people in general. Thus the teaching context embodies both the uniqueness of this moral intuition and the implication of its availability to other such cases. This is so because the learning of a moral word is the learning of a rule for its use. Like the tacit rule of grammar that allows for the generation of an infinity of well-formed sentences, the tacit rule for the use of a moral intuition allows for the generation of an infinity of conventionally well-formed moral intuitions.[5]

There is also a more pregnant social use of example in the context of human moral education. Persons, their actions, and their personalities can be examples, too. The heroes, saints, and great persons of any society become moral exemplars for the young of that society. Their actions and personalities are taken to embody just the kind of action and personality traits thought to be good and right. It is a graphic mark of the social character of morality that children and even adults are often advised to use someone else's behavior as a model for their own; not, of course, in the strict sense of literally doing just what another has done, but in the wider sense of doing something like what the admired person has done. Such persons themselves embody ideals of human conduct. The uniqueness of their personalities and activities becomes a rule for the generation of an indefinite number of similar personalities and activities. In the many moral intuitions of other persons generated by reflection on such moral exemplars, the self-transcending connection between ideal and fact in morality becomes manifest: The earnest moral conscience asks itself how its ideal person would respond in these circumstances and factually does so itself.

It is also true that we are often explicitly taught that a moral intuition is general and applies to all such cases as in "these things are always bad" and "these actions are always right." Morality is thus consciously univer-

46

C. Will, Virtue, and Habit

Morality is a fact of our natural and conventional experience but it is also related directly to our ideals. If values in general specify aspects of ideals and concrete intuitions of value and duty have their sources in the values we seek to attain and preserve, then all of morality will be a function of ideals. These moral ideals, like all ideals, will be vague and only half conscious in the lives of those persons and societies who act in their light. Still, moral ideals will be the controlling forces which give order and direction to persons' individual intuitions of value and duty.

This relationship to the ideal makes morality eminently practical. Ideals in general motivate us to action in order that we may more fully realize those ideals in fact, and moral ideals in particular govern our actions with respect to ourselves and to other persons. Our intuitions of value and duty salized in intent. This social character of the learning of moral intuitions and this making universal of our moral intuitions are the grounds for our ability to name similar moral situations with the same name, to judge the adequacy of our own moral intuitions and those of others, and to seek and give moral advice. This social and universalizing dimension of moral experience is learned early and with deep emotional association. It shows itself throughout human moral reasoning from the lament of the small child that so and so did it, "so why can't I?" to the chagrin of the adult at being treated differently from relevantly similar others. Further, this moral teaching and learning does not cease after childhood. Rather, it is central to all adult moral criticism. Appeal to the social and universalizing intent of morality continues so long as a person and a society continues to be open to growth through experience and reflection upon it.

It appears then to be a fact of our moral experience that it is both radically unique to its own person and circumstances and yet is bound by the social and universalizing dimensions of the teaching and learning context. The morally mature person, therefore, is compelled to respond both to each unique moral situation and to the features of those unique moral situations which make them similar to other moral situations. The exercise of moral intuition in any and all cases will exhibit this ambiguity, this tension between the unique and the similar. The well trained good sense of the morally educated individual and the earnest moral conscience which this implies is the only standard available to resolve this tension in the moment of moral intuition and of action on the basis of moral intuition. Outside of this moment in which the exigencies of action compel intuitive choice, our moral intuitions and consequent actions are constantly criticized by others and by our own temporally later selves. Thus there is a continuous interplay between the unique and the similar in moral education, in intuition and action, and in social and personal criticism. The tension of these opposing facets of morality embedded within this learning, doing, assessing, and relearning provides persons and societies with an energy and a means for ongoing moral self-transcendence.

47

introduce moral controls directly into our actions. The intuition that something is good is not only a conventional description but also, other things being equal, a command to seek that thing.[6] The intuition that something is forbidden and therefore wrong to do is not only an assertion of conventional fact but also, other things being equal, a command to refrain from that something. In general, morality not only describes facts of the social world but it also prescribes personal conduct. Thus, the value and duty intuitions of morality make it a powerful tool, a tool through which ideals enter facts and thus help remake reality.

It is a commonplace that this action implication of our moral intuitions is not always satisfied in practice. On many occasions, persons have a strongly felt intuition of value and yet do not seek to attain that value, or a strongly felt intuition of duty and yet do not perform or forbear as the intuition indicates. At times, this is because of the conflicting tugs of other strongly felt intuitions, as when the attainment of one value makes the attainment of another impossible or when duties are in an outright conflict. But there are other times in which the agent has a clear and conflict free intuition and yet fails to translate that intuition into action. This is a weakness in the will, a frailty in that aspect of a person which is the capacity for decision and action.[7] Since the function of morality is to govern action, such weakness must be reduced to a minimum in the person and in society if morality is to be successful on its own terms.

By contrast, the ability to translate moral intuition into action is correspondingly a strength of the will, or as we sometimes say, a strength of character. The production of such strength is a desideratum for morality. The most obvious way in which strength of character is produced is by the repetition of acts of will to the point of the production of a habit, a habit of routinely deciding and acting on one's moral intuitions. But there is a curious paradox here. I can only be sure of translating my intuitions into action now if I routinely translate my intuitions into action, but I can only routinely do so if I did do so in the face of the now I experienced yesterday, and I could only do so yesterday if I had done so in the now of the day before yesterday, etc. In other words, assuring strength of will here and now requires a habit of such strength, but one only has the habit of such strength if one has exercised it in a series of heres and nows in the past. This paradoxically circular character of habit formation might be sufficient grounds for the theoretical rejection of the whole notion were it not for the fact that experiences of building and unbuilding habits are part of every person's daily life. One simply must acknowledge the central role of habit in all things human. Perhaps part of the theoretical difficulty in understanding habit formation can be reduced by the observation that the whole process is begun for us before we are consciously aware of it by the genetically habituated actions of the body and by the habits of behavior imposed on us as children by our parents in particular and the adult world in general. We are born into and develop everywhere within a web of habits. Thus we do not ourselves consciously initiate any habit building or unbuilding without the prior existence of a whole panoply of unconscious habits formed in us by other persons and by society in general. Therefore, the relative weakness or strength of our individual wills begins to be shaped before we can meaningfully participate in the process.

The attainment in a person of strong habits of translating appropriate moral intuitions into actions is virtue. Virtue, therefore, is moral excellence. The virtuous person "knows" what need to be done morally and does it. This is no simple task. The production of a virtuous person is a personal and social achievement of considerable magnitude. For the virtuous person to have the appropriate intuitions means that he or she has heard the right stories, learned the right rules, adopted the right exemplars, felt the right feelings, and made the right reflective choices. It also means that he or she knows how to apply these moral lessons in novel circumstances; it means, for example, knowing intuitively when an exception to a rule is called for and when it is not, when a situation's moral uniqueness is more compelling than its moral similarity and when it is not. The virtuous person also must frequently and reliably make the decisions and perform the actions dictated by his or her moral intuitions so as to build a moral habit of strength of the will. For the virtuous person to achieve this habitual strength of will means that he or she was given the right habits initially by parents, siblings, friends, and society in general and that he or she has consciously built additional strengths on top of these inherited ones. Attainment of the moral excellence of virtue requires subtle contextual intuitions of value and duty and the unyielding habit of moving those intuitions into action.

Habit functions similarly at the societal level of morality as well. There is a routine translation of intuitions into actions through the social habits embodied in institutions and practices. A society's inability to create the institutions and practices necessary to engage its moral intuitions with action is a collective weakness of will, as in the case of a society which espouses intuitions of the value of human equality and justice but provides no social mechanisms to guarantee equal access to impartial justice. By contrast, the social structuring of institutions and practices to realize in action the moral intuitions of a society is a collective strength of character, as in the opposite case of a society which espouses intuitions of human equality and justice and does provide social mechanisms to guarantee equal access to impartial courts for all its citizens. The establishment of such habitual strength of will at the social level is of critical importance since these social habits create the moral horizon against which the next generation of persons will form their own personal habits or, more accurately, against which the early habits of the next generation of persons will be formed for them. This, in a phrase, is moral socialization: the making of new personal habits against the horizon of the received social habits.

These admissions of the central role of habit in the shaping of moral character at the personal and social levels should not blind us to the potential for negative consequences inherent in the functioning of habit. The

49

first and obvious point here is that some habits are bad ones. Persons can become habitually deceitful, selfish, and cruel; indeed, everything deemed bad and wrong can be routinely sought and done through habit. It is nearly a matter of definition that what is bad or wrong in itself is worse for becoming a habit. Obvious here too are the personal habits of moral backsliding, of grasping for a lesser present value over a greater future value, or of grasping for a value even where it conflicts with a stronger intuition of duty. Weakness of will also can become a habit, that is, one can make a habit of one's inability to form other appropriate habits. At the social level, many institutions and practices are habits we could well do without, like the institution of slavery or the practice of murdering political opponents. The negative effects of such bad social habits are multiplied through the personal habits of those who are morally socialized by these institutions and practices.

In addition, it is a matter of common experience that habits once formed are notoriously difficult to change. This too follows from the very nature of habit. If a habit just is a disposition to behave in a certain way because of the accumulated psychological and social weight of having behaved in that way with routine in the past, then the attempt to alter a habit will mean opposing this act in this moment against that accumulated weight of past acts. The common experiences of dieting, giving up cigarettes, or changing one's vocabulary and patterns of speech give sufficient evidence that breaking habits is no easy matter.

Yet such alteration in moral habits is just what is called for by the theory of reality we have described. Reality, on this account, is a combination of the fact world and the ideal world and because ideals are dynamically related to fact and vice versa, reality itself is in constant change. Our actions in light of our ideals lead to change in the facts of the world. This change in fact can lead to different perspectives on our ideals or to outright change in the ideals themselves. So if morality is the tool for the application of our ideals to the fact world through the medium of moral intuitions and acts of will, then habits of morality will have to take cognizance of changes in the worlds of fact and ideal and change themselves accordingly. In simple terms, when the facts of the world change, I had better change my habits to accord with the new facts. When the ideals of my world change, I had better change my habits to accord with the new ideals. New realities require new habits.

It is the difficulty inherent in habit change that gives rise to extreme moral conservatism. From what we have seen, it follows that commitment to morality in a changing reality requires that we carefully conserve the moral accomplishments we have inherited personally and socially by structuring these accomplishments into our personal habits and social institutions. Thus, at the very outset, we must admit a certain truth to the conservative position: We must conserve the moral achievements of the past. Nevertheless, morality will rapidly become irrelevant if it refuses to change in a changing world. Since its very success as a morality changes the world in fact and in ideal, the moral task of continuously applying ideals to facts entails that we must stay ever sensitive to changes in either or both. The extreme moral conservative sees the moral habits of his or her life and his or her society as fixed and definitive of morality as such. They may, of course, be fixed, in fact, for this person and for that society and they may, in ignorance of history and with the force of sheer dogmatism, present themselves ideally as the only conceivable moral habits. In such a situation, moral change is made impossible by fiat, by dogged tenacity to the ideals and facts of yesterday.[8] Any new moral intuitions are not taken to be moral at all from this perspective but a fall from morality to the immoral or the amoral. But a morality like this, a morality that will not change, is a morality incapable of progress. A morality incapable of progress is no morality at all since it has surrendered its central task of progressively realizing ideal in fact. Thus, the extreme moral conservative has given up the challenge of creating and recreating a living and relevant morality for the cognitive and emotional comfort of hidebound personal habits and rigid social institutions.

So while admitting the importance of habit and the truth in a certain measure of conservatism for the sake of taking the accomplishments of the past into the future; admitting this, we must still insist that the nature of reality requires close scrutiny of new facts, sensitivity to new ideals, and the willingness to exchange new habits for old. Morality needs a method of systematically renewing its own relevance, a method of keeping its intuitions of value and duty alive and growing with reality. Morality needs the periodic conscious reflections of ethics.

Chapter 5.

Ethics

A. Action and Reflection

One of the most evident facts about the experience of morality is that it presents itself as authoritative. Part of the reason for this is that morality is practical and is designed to lead to action. Action, by its nature, must be quick, sure, and emotionally satisfying to the agent if it is to be successful on its own terms; hesitation, uncertainty, and emotional frustration impair successful action. Consequently, our moral intuitions generally carry with them a sense of obviousness and conviction, a sense of authority sufficient to consolidate the self of the agent in successful action. In moral contexts, we generally act with a clear, decisive conscience and in many cases with a formed habit of so acting.

The social character of morality exhibits this characteristic of authority as well. The social institutions and practices contained within our religious traditions, legal systems, and social conventions contain highly structured public habits which provide for the generation of moral intuitions so clear and decisive as to lead in general to quick, sure, and emotionally satisfying action. Religions present their moral intuitions with the authority of divine revelation as contained in sacred writings and traditions. Legal systems, within their own jurisdictions, have authoritative moral intuitions in codified law, in the precedents of past intuitions and actions, and in the institutionalized procedures for resolving conflict and administering justice. Social conventions are so authoritative at times that they strike us with the force of nature itself. "Everybody does it" is for most people the final authority on all moral questions and for everyone the final authority on some moral questions.

As we have seen, there is need for periodic inspection of these moral authorities, of these personal and social habits. The very nature of morality demands attention to new realities and the conscious alteration of habit in light of these new realities. But there are other reasons internal to these authorities for periodic criticism of their habits. Our consciences, though usually authoritative, can sometimes be divided and confused, rendering them less than helpful as arbiters of intuition and action. Further, we know that appeal to conscience can often be self-deceptive, can be a way of providing justifications for narrow self-interest or for behavior that seeks the path of least resistance.[1] We also know now that personal conscience is strongly influenced by a host of early childhood experiences. Not only is the conscience known to be formed by parental and societal values, values which themselves may be in need of inspection, but also by such accidental and emotive happenings as early experiences of shame and fright. Personal conscience, for these reasons, may not always be a very reliable moral authority; it needs periodic inspection.

Religiously based moral authority, while the strongest in theory, is weakened in fact by the sheer plurality of religious perspectives. When one religion asserts that a moral intuition has divine authority and another asserts that it does not, the moral authority of all religion is underminded. Even internal to a single religion, a long enough historical perspective will generally reveal changes in moral intuitions of considerable importance. Further, in a secular society, while every person will still have a morality as we have defined it, not every person will identify with the authority of an organized religion. Finally, there are weighty and intractable philosophical difficulties in understanding, without a prior faith commitment, the being and nature of God, God's relationship to persons and the world, and the basis for our alleged human ability to interpret God's intentions through sacred writings and tradition.[2] Consequently, though religion has been and likely will continue to be a source and a bearer of some of our most profound moral intuitions, its own authority in these moral matters needs periodic inspection.

The law, too, differs in place and in time and dramatically so. Though the law is a powerful moral authority within its own jurisdiction, the idea that what is right in one jurisdiction can be wrong in another is confusing to the social and universalizing intent in morality. The law is also at once wider and more narrow than morality; wider in the sense that it also addresses issues that are not particularly moral in character and narrower in the sense that it does not speak to all of what we would intuitively feel as morally important. Law, for example, regulates the minutia of traffic control but cannot enforce a significant but private promise. Finally, it is clear that some societies have had and continue to have laws which are repugnant to our contemporary moral intuitions, laws allowing slavery, genocide, racism, sexism, etc. The moral authority of law, then, is itself in need of periodic inspection.

Our social conventions provide us with potentially significant moral facts when it is clear that "everybody" in a society thinks that a certain thing is good or a certain action is wrong. This consensus may express some powerful and acceptable moral intuitions at the social level. On the other hand, social conventions often differ dramatically from one society to another and can even give rise to conflicting intuitions within a single society. The moral consensus which these social conventions express can be the result of errors, false assumptions, or mindless fashions. And some societies have had and do have conventions which are also repugnant to our contemporary moral intuitions, conventions such as extremely patriarchal families, ceremorial disfigurement of the body, the driving of fast cars while intoxicated, etc. The moral authority of social conventions also needs periodic inspection.

There must, therefore, be a way for morality to periodically inspect its habitual intuitions at the personal and social levels. That way is through ethics. Ethics is the discipline of conscious reflection on morality; it is the clarification, organization, and critique of our individual and habitual intuitions of value and duty for the sake of continued moral progress. As morality is primarily the emotive and habitual experience of intuitions, so ethics is primarily the use of reason. Ethics periodically suspends the otherwise compelling authorities of morality for the sake of bringing them before the authority of reason, that is, before the authority of our personal and social experience and our conscious reflections about them. Since periodic rational inspection of morality is necessary if morality is to remain a living and relevant part of our experience, and because the authorities of morality open themselves to the problems we have described, ethical reflection is a periodic occurrence in all moralities except in the cases of the most dogmatically traditional persons and societies. In other cases, ethics is an aspect of morality. As reason is an episodically expressed aspect of our total experience, so ethics is an episodically expressed aspect of our total morality.

Ethics seeks to clarify our moral intuitions so that we can more readily see what actions these intuitions require of us. As a part of philosophy, ethics asks radical questions, questions which generate questioning and tentative answers. Do I really have this duty to this person and what are my reasons for thinking that I do? Is this confused sense I feel indicative of a conflict of value intuitions or is it a sign of the weakness of my will? Is it truly clear to me that this value is more worthy than that value, this duty more obligatory than that duty, or this value more compelling than that duty? Can I better perceive the ideals that stand obscurely behind my intuitions of value and duty? Questions like these, and the investigations which these questions generate, express the attempts of ethical reflection to clarify our moral experience.

Ethics also seeks to organize our moral intuitions to eliminate conflict and produce consistency. The organizing thrust of ethics asks questions such as these. How do my personal values and duties relate to those of my society and are they compatible? Does this specific duty to another person oblige me further as well? Does commitment to human equality entail rejection of all forms of racism and sexism? Does it require greater equalization of life opportunities? Above all, the organizing bent of ethics leads us to seek for unifying principles running throughout all of our moral intuitions. Is all of morality basically self-love, or altruism, or both? Is the maximization of human happiness the principle of all value intuitions? Is justice to others the fundamental principle of all intuitions of duty? Is the "Golden Rule" the essence of all our moral intuitions? Here, as in every use of reason's organizing ability, there is the problem of knowing whether our proposed answers to these questions are discovered or created. It will be hard to know whether these principles and others like them are truly "there" in our moral intuitions as an implied organization or whether the creative power of reason imposes them on our intuitions upon reflection. There is never a simple solution to this problem but reason seeks consistency nevertheless. And even if this consistency is created and not discovered, such creativity, if it does render our moral intuitions more consistent than initially experienced, is itself an important dimension of moral progress. It is an improvement, other things being equal, to make one's own or society's moral intuitions not only clearer but more consistent as well.

Finally, ethics seeks to critique our moral intuitions. Criticism is already implied in the acts of clarification and organization of moral intuitions, since one normally rejects or modifies unclear and inconsistent intuitions. Criticism is thus internal to the other operations of ethics but it is external as well. Ethics seeks to criticize our moral intuitions by judging their acceptability or unacceptability in light of other standards. These standards are themselves matters for reflective discussion. It is by no means clear what are the relevant standards to use in any given case and philosophers have drawn them from many diverse sources, such as religion, art, and science. But even if the specifics of the standards employed are matters in need of further justification, at least the general outline of criticism is clear. Ethics primarily criticizes moral intuitions with respect to the general standards implied in our knowledge of the fact world, our sensitivity to our ideals, and the truths we hold to be expressive of the resulting reality. Intuitions of value impossible to realize in fact are clearly unacceptable. Intuitions of duty incompatible with our conception of the best available ideals are clearly unacceptable. The criticism of ethics is thus designed to keep our moralities in touch and in active engagement with reality.

This last characteristic of ethics and the difficulties attendant to it reveal another important feature of reasoning about morality. Ethics is never complete, never finished. I may have criticized my moral intuitions in light of the best standards available only to find that I now have to criticize those standards themselves. Or I may criticize one particular moral intuition and find that later reflection uncovers new dimensions of that intuition, dimensions I had overlooked. New facts and new ideals constantly renew the need for more reflection as well. Reasoning here, as in all of its expressions, is thus contextual, episodic, and partial.

There are some other important implications about ethics suggested by this account. First, ethics is not a substitute for morality. Ethics itself cannot make persons or societies moral. The morality of any person or society is a conventionally shaped natural fact and is a pervasive characteristic of human response to the environment. The clarifications, organizations, and criticisms of ethics must presume a given moral horizon and begin its partial reformations from that standpoint. No person or society can respond to the demands of action directly in terms of ethics, since the character of reasoning, unlike that of emotion and habit, is slow, tentative, and emotionally thin. We must act on our moral intuitions constantly, even as we episodically submit some of them to the scrutiny of ethics.

A second important implication of this view of ethics is that the exclusively rational findings of ethics cannot of themselves compete with the emotional richness of morality. No rational argument alone will change a deeply felt moral intuition. Instead, ethics, while primarily rational, must also make use of the emotive energy in morality on behalf of its own reform. The rational clarification of an intuition of value also clarifies our feelings. The very drive for organized consistency in our moral intuitions is itself a powerful emotion and, when succesful, can graft one emotion on to another and thus help to make our feelings stronger and more consistent. Criticism of moral intuitions, even allegedly rational criticism, has such a patently affective dimension that many persons find it too painful and too draining an emotional experience. In some, moral emotions run so strongly that ethical criticism provokes outright hostility.[3] An ethical reflection that seeks to genuinely engage the received morality with the evolving worlds of fact and ideal will have to be cognizant of this emotional life of morality and handle it intelligently. The educated emotions of the morally mature person are an achievement, however partial, which ethics must seek to preserve into the future.

Finally, the partial and episodic character of ethical reflection entails that ethics must be redone and rethought by each person and society without ever becoming complete. But ethics does seek a goal: continued moral progress in the lives of individual persons and societies, continued progress in realizing our moral ideals in fact. Perhaps there will never be a time when such progress is brought to completion. Still the nature of the process itself allows the hope that earnest ethical reflection and earnest moral commitment, if continued indefinitely, will bring us individually and collectively ever closer to realizing in fact our ideals of autonomous persons in progressive societies — or perhaps to realizing the even finer ideals that may evolve from these. In any event, here as elsewhere, the use of reason can help to make us free, or at least freer; freer from blind obedience to the moral authority of personal and social habit and the negative practical consequences blind obedience often brings.

B. Doing Good

Let us begin ethical reflection on our moral intuitions by consideration of one of the most simple and straightforward principles ever suggested to be at the heart of morality: "Do good and avoid evil."[4] Examination of this principle can help us to clarify our moral intuitions by helping us to see which aspects of our morality are captured by this ethical principle. Since this principle has been held to be at the root of all our moral intuitions, examination of it should help us discover or create an organization among these intuitions. It may also help us criticize our morality by revealing aspects of the ideal and fact worlds which we live through but take no notice of. These ideals and facts may then provide us with standards on which to base criticism of our moral intuitions.

The first point to notice about the imperative to do good and avoid evil is that it is not redundant but in fact two separate imperatives. It is often the case that we can only do good at the cost of doing some evil. It is also often the case that we can only avoid evil at the cost of doing no good. This principle commands us to do both but provides no direction in cases of such conflict. Let us therefore divide this principle into its parts and consider them separately, taking the imperative to do good first.

Since we have already defined a moral value as a specification of an ideal, let us now define 'good.' Something is good if it is the object of an act of valuing. If I value some thing it is because I take that thing or activity to be good. Goodness, then, is a property of what I seek when I value something and my valuing of something is my act of taking it to be a good. As with the case of ideals themselves, the notions of value and good are wider than morality; all these words have both moral and nonmoral uses. I may embrace the moral value of honesty and therefore regard persons who are honest and their honest actions as morally good. I may also embrace the nonmoral, natural value of health and regard healthy persons and healthful activities as good. As these examples may suggest, the distinction between moral values and natural, nonmoral values will be hard to draw sharply. Many values will contain elements of both moral and nonmoral goods. Any moral good is capable of producing a significant nonmoral good if it makes us psychologically happy when we attain it, for example. In spite of this admission, the general distinction between moral and nonmoral goods should be clear. Some goods like honesty, respect for persons' rights, and free political institutions are moral values. These goods have to do with achievements of that aspect of our experience which is moral. Some goods like pleasure, happiness, and health are natural and nonmoral values. These goods have to do with preferred natural states.

The nonmoral goods of our lives are based on nature itself. Since our bodies are naturally attracted to pleasure and naturally repelled by pain, physical pleasure is a natural, nonmoral good and one that we spontaneously and constantly seek. The natural valuing of food, sleep, exercise, sex, warmth, etc. are facts about human beings in every society. At the same time, the natural facts of human psychology attract us to happiness and repel us from suffering. These facts make happiness in all of its many expressions a natural, nonmoral good and one spontaneously and constantly sought by human beings. By contrast, the moral values of honesty, respect for persons' rights, and free political institutions are conventional, moral, and not at all universal throughout human society.

This difference between moral and nonmoral goods and the apparently primordial character of the nonmoral ones has led some thinkers to suggest that all moral goods are primarily valuable for the nonmoral goods they can produce for us. Thus, on this account, we value honesty not for anything about honesty in itself but because honest relationships bring us considerable pleasure and happiness and they tend to minimize experiences of pain and suffering. This ethical view holds that moral goods and by implication all of the values of morality are basically instruments for the attainment of nonmoral goods. Morality, then, is useful for us; it has utility. Hence, one of the most influential ethical position associated with this perspective is called utilitarianism. It emphasizes the doing of good over the avoidance of evil and it sees all moral goods as valuable for the nonmoral goods they can produce.[5] Since the primary nonmoral goods are the natural experiences of pleasure and happiness, utilitarian ethics urges us to always choose to do whatever will maximize the resultant amount of pleasure and happiness over the amount of pain and suffering or, where pleasure and happiness cannot be maximized, to minimize the amount of pain and suffering directly. The utilitarian also insists on the social and universalizing intent of morality so that the pleasure and happiness sought is not solely that of the agent but of all those involved who are capable of feeling pleasure and pain, happiness and suffering. This ethical theory thus commits one to the use of moral goods (e.g. honesty) for the purpose of producing for all involved the greatest amount of nonmoral goods (e.g. happiness). Let us say for short that utilitarian ethics demands that we maximize happiness.

Utilitarianism is a powerful ethical theory. It clarifies the nature of our moral intuitions. It gives these intuitions systematic organization. It affords a clear and meaningful standard for the criticism of personal and social habits of moral intuition and action: Do these intuitions and the actions they direct maximize happiness or not? If the answer is negative, utilitarianism can propose new intuitions which will be surer producers of happiness. The use of this theory at the personal level can make an individual's moral life more clear, orderly, and self-critical. Its use at the social level can provide a readily intelligible instrument for the criticism and change of bad social institutions and practices.[6] And utilitarianism seems to be true to much of our physical and psychological experience: Persons do seek the nonmoral goods of pleasure and happiness.

There are several serious objections to this ethical theory, however. When it was initially proposed in a manner which emphasized the goal of attaining pleasure exclusively, it was branded the "philosophy of a pig."[7] The point behind this rhetorical flourish was that utilitarianism in this form too much emphasized the role of the body and reduced the dignity of all human moral strivings to the level of an animal's drive for sense pleasure. The utilitarian principle was subsequently expanded in light of this criticism to include the richer concept of happiness. This expanded version of utilitarianism is not so vulnerable to this criticism, but it too tends to rob our moral life of any significance in and of itself. Morality is still seen to be purely an instrument for the production of nonmoral goods. One might suppose on this account that if there were other nonmoral but equally useful means of producing the same amount of happiness produced now by morality, then the moral dimension of our lives could be replaced by these nonmoral means without loss. Suppose, for example, that certain chemicals could induce long-standing feelings of happiness, feelings free of any negative consequences. Would morality then be irrelevant? Suppose these chemicals made us inevitably maximize happiness for all involved. Would morality then be replaced? One feels that there is more to morality than this, that morality has some significance in and of itself, even if it is often directly related to our search for happiness. In sum, the thrust of this first criticism is that utilitarianism wrongly ignores the direct human significance of moral goods themselves, the importance to us, in themselves, of being certain kinds of persons and doing certain kinds of actions.

Associated with this point is the further objection that utilitarianism is simply too radical a revision of our moral intuitions to accept as an adequate ethical theory. Certainly, we do not usually regard our moral values as wholly related to the search for happiness. When faced with a moral problem, we seldom reduce it wholly to the question of what action maximizes happiness. While utilitarianism does help us to clarify, organize, and critique our moral intuitions, it also seems to change them in a quite wholesale fashion. It would appear that in many situations, the application of this principle directly would result in intuitions in conflict with some of what are now our most securely felt intuitions. A murder, for example, could be permitted, could even be obligatory, if the net gain in happiness was large enough. The same point can be made about lying, torture, infidelity, stealing, and about all of the fundamental intuitions of our conventional morality. The radical character of utilitarianism's revision of our moral intuitions becomes even more plain if one asks if this view ought to be taught to children. Would one teach a child that morality is only about nonmoral happiness making or would this insight be preserved for adults? Should one teach children that murder is wrong unless it can maximize happiness and then it is right or even obligatory? The distance from our received moral intuitions here seems too great for utilitarianism to be accepted as a reflective interpretation of our morality.[8] These considerations make it appear that utilitarianism is really being offered as a replacement morality. If it is being proposed as a replacement for our inherited morality, the question we must ask is why we should accept such a wholesale replacement. Our present habits of experiencing and acting on moral intuitions, in spite of their numerous inadequacies, are products of a long historical development and thus have largely proved their worth in the crucible of generations of daily life. What are the grounds for thinking that we need such a radical revision? This seems to be a case in which the creative dimension of reason's organizing tendencies has too far outstripped its discovery dimension. Utilitarianism makes of morality a very coherent and orderly system, but it seems not to be the morality we know through experience.

Additional difficulties arise with the use of the theory. Since it commands that we perform that action which will maximize happiness, it is presumed by the utilitarian that we can know or discover which action that is. But such happiness consequences are in the future, and the future is what it is by virtue of the fact that it is an unknown, a field of open possibilities. Of course, it is true that it is the task of reasoning generally to plan for the future. As such, rational persons everywhere make reasonable assumptions about what the character of the future is likely to be. We all plan for tomorrow without exaggerated intellectual doubts about what that tomorrow will be like. Yet we do make mistakes; our plans do go awry. The future as it becomes present often reveals consequences of our actions that we could never have anticipated and planned for. An ethical theory which places all of its emphasis on future consequences must acknowledge this lack of knowledge, this ability of tomorrow to take us by surprise. This point has practical bearing. To move, for example, from the traditional moral claim that this act of murder is wrong to the revised claim that this act of murder may be right or wrong depending upon what pleasures and happinesses tomorrow brings introduces considerable difficulties into the context of choice and action. Not only then has utilitarianism reduced the moral to the nonmoral but it has also replaced the moral surety of today with reference to the possibilities of tomorrow, possibilities about which we may be wholly mistaken. How many times has each of us transgressed moral convention for the sake of securing some future happiness only to find that unhappiness was the result? Consider the extreme case of an assassin whose murder of a political tyrant brings a reign of worse terror instead of the political freedoms sought. Our moral choices may seldom be so dramatic but they share with this case the real imponderability of the future. Utilitarianism relies on future knowledge, knowledge we can never have securely.

There are problems, too, in determining the nature of happiness. Pleasure as a natural fact is far more universal and palpable than happiness but, as the charge of being a "philosophy of a pig" indicates, it is also far less acceptable as the basis of an ethical theory. The shift to expand utilitarianism to include the richer notion of happiness introduces all of the ambiguities of that notion into the ethical theory itself. It is a fact of life that what brings happiness to one person and society does not necessarily bring happiness to other persons and societies. What are we to do with those whose happiness seems to lie in immoral behavior itself, in crime, or in the infliction of pain on others? Furthermore, there is a growing number of reasons to think that our experiences of pleasure and happiness are indefinitely plastic.[9] Changes in our genetic inheritance, whether conscious or not, could well provoke changes in what gives the body pleasure and the mind happiness. More obviously, behavior conditioning, again whether consciously or not, can make marked changes in what makes for happiness. The mass media, for example, has made it hard for persons in developed nations to be happy without a whole range of consumer goods not even in existence a century ago. Such dramatic examples of conditioning aside, what makes for human happiness presents endless variety. The happiness some find in personal freedom brings others only the sufferings of loneliness and confusion. The happiness some find in the social cohesion of small towns and rural life brings others only frustration and a sense of being stifled. For some, happiness is an endless pursuit of exhilaration and stimulation; for others, tranquility and relaxation. Which happiness should we seek to maximize, and how are we to manage all of these variables in the context of moral choice? The utilitarian ethical theory gives us no direction here.

Finally, utilitarianism has a problem with justice and the recognition of the rights of individual persons. An overall increase in the net amount of happiness can often be had at the expense of the sufferings of the few. In fact, one can conceive of situations, such as the slavery of a minority racial or ethnic group, in which the maximization of total happiness can only be had because the sufferings of some bring happiness to many. So long as the miserable are few and the happiness for the many is great, the mathematics of happiness maximization will run over the rights of the individual person and of small groups of persons. This same point can be made temporally as well. A violation of the rights of a few today may be mandatory according to this view if the indefinite generations of humans to follow are all counted as beneficiaries of this violation. Perhaps we could eliminate forever certain genetic diseases and all the sufferings they cause by putting today's carriers to death. Maybe the vivisection of a few persons today could improve our medical care of all human persons to follow and thus maximize happiness over time. What are your rights and mine compared to the total happiness of all human beings who come after us? The implied quantification in this ethical theory is thus a threat to the single individual or small group. And it offends our sense of justice, that very strong moral intuition of duty towards others that makes us "know" these acts would be wrong even if they did maximize happiness.

For these reasons, utilitarianism is not acceptable as the definitive ethical theory. Yet this view still has force, the very force of our physical and psychological natures. This truth in utilitarianism must be taken up into any more adequate theory. Surely morality has something to do with our drives for pleasure and happiness, even if we have now found the complete reduction of the moral to the nonmoral to be unacceptable.

C. Avoiding Evil

Concentration on the second part of our principle, do good and avoid evil, will provide us with a different perspective. Evil, of course, is what we take to be bad, the negative correlative of good. What is evil is the opposite of what we value; something from which we are normally repelled. The most obvious evils are the nonmoral evils of pain and suffering, those states of our bodies and our minds that we most want to avoid. But there are moral evils as well. Murder, lying, torture are examples of clear moral evils.

If we take the suggestion implied by our rejection of utilitarianism, the suggestion that moral goods are not merely instrumental for the production of nonmoral goods; if we take this suggestion, the relevant implication here is that the moral evils of action like murder, lying, and torture are not merely in their abilities to produce the nonmoral evils of pain and suffering. Moral evils can do that too, of course. Murder can cause physical pain to the victim and suffering to loved ones left behind. Lying can cause great suffering and, through its consequences, even physical pain. Torture and the many other obvious moral evils similarly cause pain, suffering, or both. This pain and suffering must be a part of why these actions are morally evil. But if our doubts about the direct connection between moral goods and the production of the nonmoral goods of pleasure and happiness are justified, then we must have similar doubts about directly connecting moral evil with the production of the nonmoral evils of pain and suffering. There must be a more central moral dimension to these evils, a moral dimension not to be reduced to the nonmoral. There must be something more wrong with murder, lying, and torture; something more than the pains and sufferings that they cause.

Perhaps that more central moral dimension of wrongness lies in the incompatibility of these actions with the central moral ideal we have already developed, the ideal of personal autonomy. If so, it will be additional confirmation of the choice of this ideal and its associated social ideal, since these ideals will help us to provide a reflective account of the evil of morally evil things and, by implication, of the good of morally good things. It surely is a fact that all of these acts are assaults on the human person's. Murder denies the person his or her very self. Lying distorts the person's grip on reality and compromises the ability to be free and rational. Torture is a direct attack on the body and mind of a person. Other evils less directly related to the person such as infidelity and stealing may be similarly analyzed by observing that persons extend themselves into their personal relationships and properties and thus may be indirectly assaulted through compromise of their personal extensions. Not only, then, do these evils cause the nonmoral evils of pain and suffering, but they do so through the moral evil of assaulting human persons.

The moral evil in assaults in the human person follows from the value which we have seen attaches to the self of the autonomous person.[10] The autonomous person is an incalculably worthy being because the self of the person is the existential point from which value is created. The person, then, is a consummate value because the self of each person is a creator of values. The person, because of this value creative activity of the self, is absolute in worth, the value of values. Assault on the person then is not merely an assault on value but on the value of values, on human dignity as the absolute value. Thus, as wrong as it is to subvert the values of pleasure and happiness by the infliction of pain and suffering, it is that much more wrong to subvert the value of values by direct assault on the human person.

As we have also seen, this incalculable value, this dignity of the person, gives rise to the notion of rights. If I am such a being with dignity, I have a right to be treated in a manner consistent with this dignity. The peculiar moral evil in murder, lying, torture, and the like, then, is that in addition to causing the nonmoral evils of pain and suffering, they violate the moral rights of persons, rights which ought to be acknowledged and respected.

If there are rights that ought to be respected, then it is wrong not to respect them. We have, then, a duty to respect persons' rights. Thus duty, the moral category exhibited in moral intuitions couched in terms of 'right' and 'wrong', is significantly related to value. Duty is our felt need to respect the value of values as the absolutely worthy source of all values. Our intuitions of duty toward ourselves and toward others are intuitive recognitions of the rights of the person, rights grounded in the dignity of the person as creator of value. Duty, therefore, is derived from value temporally and yet precedes it in moral importance. Duty derives from value temporally because only when one has experienced empirically the attractiveness of value and considered its source in the value creative activity of the human self does one have the key for understanding the nature of duty. Duty precedes value morally since the attractiveness of the source of all value must be inherently more attractive than any given value or set of values. Thus, we experience value first in time, even as we first experience the pleasures and happinesses of our bodies and our minds. But we experience duty as first morally, even as we forsake pleasures and happinesses which can only be had by assaults on the rights of persons.

This point has a social and historical expression as well. All human societies throughout history have had and do have values. Persons of every human society at all times have found certain goods inherently attractive both naturally and morally. All human societies throughout history have had and do have a sense of duty as well, but the completion of this sense of duty in the acknowledgement of and respect for human rights is not nearly universal. Consciousness of human rights and the dignity of the person are late moral developments, developments with important historical anticipations, of course, but late moral developments nevertheless.[11] The concept of rights appears not to have played any significant moral or political role in ancient or early medieval society.[12] The conceptual framework needed for the notion begins perhaps as early as ancient Stoicism and the natural law theories of the medievals, but specific recognition of the value centrality of the human person and the rights consequent upon that recognition evolved slowly in western morality. It was not until the intellectual ferment which preceded the modern democratic revolutions in England (1688), America (1776), and France (1789) that the notion of the rights of the human person became a reasonably clear and socially dynamic moral concept.[13] It was also approximately at this time that the companion social ideal of progressive societies began to be articulated in ideal and to become influential in fact. In the twentieth century, the notion of human rights has moved considerably from the ideal world of eighteenth century manifestos into the factual world of legal codes, international agreements, and progressive social habits for the protection and enhancement of human rights. As imperfect a reality as this remains today, we may still count this as moral progress if the duty to recognize rights is the morally central insight that this account suggests.

At this point, we can clarify an earlier claim that value is progressive and duty conservative. Human persons and societies have discovered and created, and likely will continue to discover and create, a myriad of values in their individual and collective experiences. New objects and activities or new perspectives on old objects and activities are constantly entering our experience as goods to value. As we strive to attain these goods, especially the moral goods among them, we develop and expand our moral consciousness and our systems of morality. The advent of worldwide mass communications adds dramatic new energy to this development and expansion. This is the dynamism of value intuitions, the dynamism of the very attraction of goodness in all of its variety. While the last several centuries have witnessed unheralded evil and developed the potential for even worse, they have also seen a growing awareness of the human person as the value of values in our personal and social habits. In view of our ideals, this has to be counted as moral progress. It has been marked by the end of legal slavery; by the guarantee of rights of personal liberty and access to necessary goods and services in several societies and the promise of these rights in others; and by significant beginnings on the road to the liberation of women, children, racial and ethnic minorities, and of other groups which have been oppressed or traditionally excluded from full participation in society.

But as we work towards and hope for the continuation of such moral development and expansion in the future, we must also conserve the value achievements of the past. One way to do this is to build an earnest moral commitment to these values into our personal and social habits. When the values at stake are absolute and incalculable as these are, our need to preserve them is felt as a strong intuition of duty, an intuition to acknowledge this dignity of persons and to respect their rights. Consequently, respect for the value of values can become an inhibitory and conservative force within the dynamic movement of value attraction. Even where there are important and highly attractive values to be had, we have a duty to refrain from having them if they involve an assault on the higher value of the person. The person from this perspective may then be considered to be both the obligatory value and the highest valued duty of our moral experience. In this light, we should alter our general principle to say: first, avoid evil, then do good; first avoid violating persons' rights, then seek other values.

We can expand and concretize this principle if we bring some of these implications back to our discussion of utilitarianism. A major flaw in that theory, as has been argued, is its reduction of moral value to nonmoral value, its equation of goodness with happiness. If moral evil is now seen to include not only the nonmoral evils of pain and suffering, but also the specifically moral, and therefore worse, evil of assault on human dignity through violation of the rights of persons, a similar result should be applied to the utilitarian ethical insight that we ought to maximize the attainment of good. Moral good, then, is not merely the attainment of pleasure and happiness, but is also and more importantly the promotion of the autonomy of persons. We value friendship and loyalty and courage, for example, not only because they can bring pleasure and happiness, but also because these activities and experiences can help make persons who are ideally free and rational more factually free and rational. Thus, the ethical insight of maximizing good is not lost, but is taken into the larger framework of an ethical commitment to satisfy the value interests of the whole person, the body that feels nonmoral pleasures, the mind that experiences nonmoral happinesses, and especially the moral consciousness that is capable of appreciating itself as the value of value continually transcending itself in ideal and fact. Furthermore, unlike utilitarianism, this entire good maximizing concern is bounded by the prior duty to avoid the moral evils inherent in assaults on human persons' rights.

Most of the flaws we indicated in utilitarianism are thus overcome. Since we value the specifically moral good of human autonomy along with the other but lesser nonmoral goods of pleasure and happiness, our theory does not wholly reduce the moral to the nonmoral. Addition of a central role for the moral good of human autonomy makes this theory far less revisionary of our received moral conventions, since the attainment of goods which might promote happiness by assault on human autonomy is forbidden on this account. The ambiguities of the meaning of happiness are now absorbed by the more general ambiguity of our ideals of autonomous persons in progressive societies and their relationships to fact; no improvement itself, perhaps, but at least a relocation of the real ambiguity of morality where it ought to be, viz., internal to morality itself. The question of our knowledge of what tomorrow will bring is not so pressing an issue for this theory, since the adjudication of many moral issues will not be deferred for tomorrow's happiness consequences but instead will be seen to be good or bad, right or wrong in the here and now by virtue of their implications for human rights. Violations of rights will be wrong as such without regard for tomorrow's happiness. Finally, the problems of utilitarianism with justice are not problems for a theory which incorporates into itself concern for the individual rights of the person as value of values.

Our own ethical principle can now be stated with some precision. One should always choose that course of action which will tend to most enhance: first, the attainment of practical personal autonomy and secondly, the attainment of happiness and pleasure for all those persons involved, but with the prior constraint of respect for the rights of all individual persons. Alternately put, one should always seek to maximize satisfactions of the moral then the nonmoral value interests of persons within the constraints of duty. Do the full range of human good; but first, avoid evil. Since the maximization of practical personal autonomy through conservation of persons' rights and through active enhancement of autonomy is the central moral notion here, this view can be entitled an ethics of autonomy maximization. Since achieving such a maximization will require considerable social as well as personal effort, this ethic conforms with our previously described ideals. Under the periodic rational control of this ethical view, morality can become a true utility: useful in serving the broadest interests of autonomous persons in progressive societies.

65

Chapter 6.

The Person as Obligatory Value

A. The Golden Rule

The category of value has a certain self-evidence since the fact of being attracted to persons, objects, or activities is a palpable dimension of the lives of all persons and societies. In fact, many of our moral problems arise just because of the strength of our value intuitions, because we are too strongly attracted to persons, objects, or activities. Thus, little more needs to be said of this obvious part of our moral consciousness. On the other hand, the category of duty is not nearly so self-evident. What is duty and how are we to know what we are duty bound to do and to refrain from? We do have a sketchy first response already: duty is the felt need to respect persons' rights. This beginning needs to be further elaborated if we are to substantiate our claim for the moral priority of duty over value and thus render a large dimension of the ethics of autonomy maximization more plausible.

The first prerequisite for understanding the general nature of duty and the concrete intuitions of duty that we experience is an examination of what we have called an earnest moral conscience. When we act with such a conscience, we are sincerely concerned to do what is right and to avoid what is wrong. We act with the best of intentions, with a good will.[1] One feature of the earnest moral conscience that stands out on reflection is the peculiar deference we pay to choice and action issuing from it even when we feel that wrong instead of right has been done. When we know that an agent sincerely intended to do right, we tend to count that intention nearly as much, perhaps more, than the actually doing of right or wrong itself. That he or she "meant well", if true, is usually sufficient to excuse the fault of having done wrong. There is a practical limit to such an excuse, of course. If a person continually insists that he or she sincerely meant to do what was right but always or often does what we take to be wrong, the suspicion will grow that this person's conscience is flawed in some way; flawed perhaps in the knowledge of right and wrong or in strength of will, but perhaps also in sincerity. Because the excuse of having had good intentions is so universally powerful, it is also subject to abuse by some persons on some occasions. Nevertheless, we are initially inclined to accept such an excuse because of the moral importance of good intentions and, of course, because the unpredictabilities of the fact world often do subvert the best of our intentions into actions judged to be wrong.

The same point about our moral consciousness can be reversed as well. Action which is right is taken to have little moral importance when it has issued from a malign or even less than earnest moral conscience. Producing a right act when one intended to do wrong or producing a right act accidently, with no intention at all; in such cases little or no moral merit accues to the agent.[2] The presence of an earnest moral conscience thus can be a powerful excuse for wrongdoing and its absence can neutralize or lessen the perceived rightness of an act.

This apparent fact about an earnest moral conscience is less surprising if one considers it to be virtually equivalent to the sense of duty itself. It may be true that there are times when sincerity of intent is necessary when dealing with values, as in a choice between two great goods or two great evils. But even in such cases, this earnestness is lightened considerably by a sense of creativity, a sense that a sincerely made value choice will tend to confirm itself by our continued embrace of it, whether or not the value choice was somehow right or wrong in itself.[3] By contrast, the earnest moral conscience approaches duty with the felt need to do what is right in itself as if the moral world contained an objective right and wrong in it. The earnest value conscience seeks to create a good choice, but the earnest duty conscience seeks to discover the right choice. In this sense, then, the earnest moral conscience is nearly equivalent to the felt need to do one's duty as one "sees" it, as objectively as one can see it.

Another way to conceive of this objective intent of an earnest moral conscience is to understand duty as an attempt to make one's choices follow moral law. Law in all of its expressions seeks to be objective. A law of nature, the law of gravity for instance, describes an objective tendency of natural objects to act in a certain consistently predictable fashion. Other things being equal, an unsupported weight descends to the surface of the earth. When other things are not equal, as with airplanes, helicopters, and rockets, we are generally capable of providing another law-like explanation of why this phenomena appears to, but does not, violate a natural law. Similarly, in the more prescriptive context of governmental legislation, a law prescribes behavior for all persons falling under a certain objective category, such as the law that, other things being equal, all automobile drivers must stop at red traffic lights. Again in this context, when other things are not equal, as in the case of emergency vehicles, legislation generally makes a law-like exception to the law; all motorists must stop at red traffic lights except in cases of bona fide emergency. Thus, the apparent violation of the law is only apparent; in fact it is governed by another law. By contrast with these law-like activities, consider the descriptive confusion that would result in science if we were content to say that airplanes violate the law of gravity and we do not know the reason why. Or consider the prescriptive confusion created at intersections if some vehicles were not required to stop at red lights without a clear reason. In these cases of law, phenomena are organized so as to account or provide for some measure of objective consistency in their behavior.

This suggests that the very nature of law is such that it treats alike what objectively is alike. Putting the point negatively, law forbids arbitrariness, forbids the treating differently of what is alike. If this is the nature of all law, then a felt duty to obey a moral law would mean the felt moral duty to treat alike what is alike. Negatively, it would mean the moral duty to avoid being arbitrary. Since morality is primarily about our actions regarding persons, commitment in duty to a moral law entails a felt need to treat alike all persons who are alike, to refrain from being arbitrary in dealings with persons. The common feeling of moral outrage exhibited in the face of arbitrary treatment is evidence in experience for this result.

Thus, there are two features of duty in a curious tension. On the one hand, there is a great deference to the earnest moral conscience, the conscience which sincerely seeks to do right even if in fact it does wrong. This deference is an expression of the subjectivity or internality of morality. Every person must choose to do what he or she earnestly believes to be the right thing to do in a unique set of circumstances. On the other hand, duty also binds us to the structure of all moral law; that is, to the non-arbitrary treating alike of what really is alike. This demand of duty is the objectivity or externality of morality. Persons must be treated the same in similar circumstances. This very tension is carried by the etymology of autonomy. The self (**auto**) must choose, but its choice must be law-like (**nomos**) in character. Thus, the freedom at the heart of autonomous choice is not the freedom of caprice and license, but the freedom of a rational, that is, lawlike choice. These two poles of morality also mirror what we have already noted about the unique and yet social and universalizing intent of moral choice. My choice is radically my own, and yet I feel that everyone faced with my situation should choose as I now choose. Indeed, this is the characteristic defense of a moral choice when its adequacy is challenged by another: Had you been in the circumstances I was in, you would have chosen as I did choose. This tension between the subjective and the objective seems to be an inevitable part of our moral conscience.

The need to address both of these poles of morality suggests an ethical reformulation of the moral demands of duty. One discharges duty only when he or she can earnestly believe that any other duty bound person in relevantly similar circumstances factually should have, and ideally would have, done the same thing. Immanuel Kant called a similar claim the categorical imperative because it expresses itself as a command of duty on all occasions without qualification.[4] This imperative does not entail that all human action will appear to be similar to the casual observer. The fact world still presents such an array of changing circumstances that many actions will be and will appear to be unique. But this duty does bind each of us to earnestly believe that what is right for me is right for all persons in like circumstances; what is wrong for me is wrong for all persons in like circumstances. It binds us to refrain from arbitrary behavior in our dealings with persons, including ourselves. Thus, we have a test by which we can help to determine our concrete duties. Can I earnestly believe that all other persons in these circumstances factually should, and ideally would, do as I am about to do? If the answer is "no," the chances are good that a duty is about to be transgressed.

68

The fact that this conclusion is remarkably similar to the traditional "Golden Rule" and that such a rule under various formulations has been a centerpiece of so many great moral traditions counts as additional confirming evidence for our ethical position.[5] We are bound to act towards others as we would have them act towards us because this is an insight into the very heart of duty. For most people, it takes little moral experience or ethical reflection to drive them to value themselves. The widespread fault of selfishness is sufficient testimony to this spontaneous self-love. The point of the "Golden Rule" is that since duty binds us to be nonarbitrary in our treatment of all persons, and since we naturally have high standards for the appropriate treatment of our own selves, the treating of other persons as we would treat ourselves guarantees both nonarbitrariness and high standards in our treatment of other persons. In our terms, the "Golden Rule" asserts that one has a duty to treat other persons with the same deference one has or should have to oneself as an incalculably worthy value of values. In both cases, incalculable value is found in the self and this value is then conferred on all other persons by the essential duty to be nonarbitrary.

There is a major presumption built into this ethical position, a presumption which becomes clear when the balance this view prescribes between the unique and the similar is challenged by the reassertion of the radically unique character of moral choice. This dimension of uniqueness follows, as we have seen, not only from the changing circumstances within which moral choice occurs, but also because of the differences among the selves who choose. If I am radically different from you, I cannot choose as you would choose. If I am radically different from you, I will demand that I be considered and treated differently. Suppose, for example, that I am better than you. Perhaps I am a master and you a slave; I am of a preferred race and gender and you are not; or I am simply and frankly a superior person.[6] Such considerations, if acceptable, could destroy our principle at its root. The theory of autonomy maximization simply cannot accept elitist claims. Consequently, these challenges indicate that there is a powerful presumption of moral equality built into this view. Our behaviors, virtues, and wills are not factually equal, but we are moral equals in the ideal sense that we are each incalculably worthy values of value. What is right for me is therefore right for you and vice versa.

Now it is a fact that human persons are seldom factually equal in any empirically measurable sense. In strength, in beauty, in intelligence, and in factual moral achievement, we all differ. Therefore, we must be presuming an ideal sense of equality, an equality not empirically measurable. Thus, we are not asserting a human equality capable of factual calculation. To express this point mathematically, each person's worth in a given respect could be assigned a natural number, as we do, for example, in I.Q. testing. Seldom are people identical in these numbers and even when they are, surely they will differ if we number every factual skill. Ideally, however, there are only two "numbers" which could make us really equal and thus could express mathematically the commitment of our ethical theory: if we were all zeroes or infinities in our ideal worth. This suggests that we can be equal only if we appraise our ideal values as persons as nothing or as infinitely great. But the very having of intuitions of duty and value and the arguments we have already seen about the value creative activity of the self exclude the first possibility. We must have some ideal moral value since we take our moralities and ourselves seriously. Therefore, if we must have some value, and that value must be presumed to be equal for all persons, then the ideal value of each person must be considered to be infinite, or in other terms, incalculably great.

Thus, this ethical principle of duty conforms with our earlier findings and further clarifies our ideals of autonomous persons in progressive societies. Though duty binds the drive to attain value by establishing the prior constraint of doing no evil to persons, it does so only because it arises out of a profound respect for the most incalculably great value of our natural experience: each human person as the value of values. The practical moral expression of this profound respect is personal and social commitment to the nonarbitrary treatment of persons, to respect for their individual rights.

B. Radical Equality and Special Rights

Our intuitive sense of moral duty leads us on ethical reflection to the ideal self of each human person as the creator of value and thus as the value of value. There is a radical equality implied here, as has been shown. Since each self is the ideal center from which the internal world of each person is constituted, each self functions similarly as a subjective value creator. Because this center of value creation is private except to each person's own introspection, there can be no direct comparisons of the relative functioning of each self in this role. Indirectly, however, we can observe in most cases the characteristically human valuing of persons, objects, activities, etc. in the lives of other persons and we are thus led to the reasonable presumption of equality on this score. Certainly, we have no nonarbitrary means of ranking the value of value creation in the lives of various persons. Cases in which such ranking has been imposed by social convention or by individual fiat as in slavery, aristocracy, sexism, or in extremely exploitative personal relationships; these cases increasingly strike the contemporary moral conscience as arbitrary and morally repugnant to our sense of duty. The very idea of buying and selling enslaved members of a racial minority as if they were merely commodities in an open market is now horrifying. The establishment of a person's rights and privileges on the basis of nobility of lineage now appears wildly arbitrary by contemporary moral standards. The idea of excluding women from full participation as equal persons in all aspects of society is also becoming increasingly repugnant to today's earnest moral conscience. The value creative activities of all racial groups, social classes, and women are too obvious to the contemporary moral sensibility to consider racism aristocracy, and sexism as anything but morally arbitrary and therefore as violations of moral duty. Increasingly, the moral burden of proof is falling on those who would treat any persons differently to prove beyond a reasonable doubt why this different treatment should not be considered arbitrary and wrong. This extension of the presumption of being equal as a person is a mark of moral progress, a progress that has taken the West from the Hellenic conception of the free, white, wellborn male as the only genuine person to the would-be democratic societies of today.[7] Our ideal of the person has developed and expanded.

Contemporary scientific and humanistic perspectives on the human person suggest an ethical goal for this moral advance: acknowledgement of membership in the human species itself as the widest, most progressive definition of the person. We know scientifically that persons are only what they are by virtue of their individual genetic inheritance. But we also know that this specific genetic inheritance is just a specification of the range of DNA formations scientifically definitive of the human species, including here a range of characteristically human mutations and defects. This species genetic material is so obviously a collective achievement of the human race that it is often and unconsciously characterized as a collectivity in the phrase, the "gene pool." Thus, the possibility of human individuation relies on the prior availability of a human genetic collectivity.

The human sciences and the humanities themselves are more and more sensitive to the role of culture in the socialization of the individual person. Culture is itself a collective human achievement made possible not only by the outstanding individual, such as the great classical violinist, but also by all of the men and women who lead more ordinary lives; by the violin maker, the trader in lumber, the lumberjack, and the forester. The achievements of culture are made possible and carried by all the various work and play activities of a society from the great to the small. Even reason and its liberating power for the person is a social achievement passed on to the individual through education and other institutionalized social habits. In short, the individual human person as value of values is a product of the physical and intellectual developments of the whole human species. As such, it seems fitting that we should establish as the reflective goal of moral progress the recognition of the equal and incalculably great value of every member of the human species as defined by the best available scientific description. Thus, the goal suggested here is that every human being should be considered a human person.

Acceptance of this logic entails that every human being is in ideal an incalculably valuable human person whether he or she factually exhibit value creative activities or not. One clear implication of this moral goal for contemporary medicine is that human beings at the "margins" of these value creative activities, beings such as the fetus, the comatose, and the severely handicapped are human persons too, and of incalculable, thus equal, value. This ethical perspective does not of itself solve the many difficult moral problems raised by the care of such categories of persons since there are generally other persons' rights at stake as well. In the case of abortion, for instance, this ethical view only serves to increase our dif-

71

ficulties, since the woman involved clearly has the same value in ideal that we have claimed for the fetus and more value in fact because of the web of real value creative activities of which she is the source. Nevertheless, the logic of moral progress suggests that these are difficulties which we will have to face earnestly and which cannot be resolved by the morally arbitrary act of reading these categories of human beings out of the ideal community of human persons.[8]

In other terms, an extension of the category of human persons is an extension of the range of human rights since respect for the person concretely entails respect for his or her rights. Since recognition of the incalculable value of the human person is the ground for our felt duty to respect persons' rights, and since all persons are of equal value, human rights by their very nature are equal. The rights of all human persons are ideally the same and are held by all human persons. The practical goal of all human rights is the same: to protect and enhance the ideal human autonomy of each human person in fact. The recognition of all human beings as possessed of equal rights will tend to insure the widest, most progressive protection and enhancement of ideal human autonomy in fact.

From a factual perspective, of course, we have to admit a great diversity in the realization of this ideal, all the way from those societies recognizing no human rights, to those recognizing some, to those with a fairly complete recognition of rights, at least in theory. Indeed, not only do the facts of the case demand this admission, but our very claims for historical progress and hope for its continuance demand that this should be so. In ideal, all human persons have equal human rights. In fact, many, even most, persons do not enjoy their rights. The distance between ideal and fact establishes the outlines of our moral goals and duties.

A cautionary note on judging other persons and societies may be appropriate here. Our ideals, when reflected upon, give us a tolerably clear picture of what actions are right and wrong. It was wrong that persons and societies countenanced and practiced slavery. It is wrong that persons and societies countenance and practice sexism. These judgments follow from our theory of duty and the central value of the human person. On the other hand, it is clear that for many of the persons and societies, perhaps most, who committed and commit these wrongs, it was and is factually impossible for them to have recognized these practices as wrong. In these societies, such practices were and are a part of the social habits against which horizon individual consciences were and are formed. If it is factually impossible for these persons and societies to see that their practices are wrong, they cannot be blamed morally.[9] Perhaps persons in these societies have the most earnest of moral consciences factually possible for them to have and still they cannot recognize the wrongness in these activities, a wrongness so palpable to us. More than any other consideration, this excuse from individual blame on the basis of the social habits of one's society underscores the need for constant criticism and progressive change of social habits. Our ideals condemn these social habits even as our sense of fact excuses the agents. Continued moral progress requires that we criticize and condemn practices incompatible with our ideals. It also makes it most inevitable that persons of the future exercising ideals we have helped to shape will roundly and rightfully condemn practices which we are factually incapable of seeing as wrong at the present.

There is another manner in which the press of the fact world must alter our ideal claims about the equality of all human rights. If the practical goal of respect for human rights is the protection and enhancement of human autonomy, then when the facts indicate that there are special threats to human autonomy at hand special rights arise.[10] This is not to say that additional rights are created, but that the general aim of equal human rights in the ideal is made particular in a factually threatening context. Such contexts are usually highly structured human relationships whose dimensions are so similar one to another and so open to assaults on human autonomy by their very natures that one can specify with some reliability the likely assaults and the measures needed to prevent them.

These special situations usually arise when human relationships are so unequal in power that the less powerful party is factually vulnerable before the more powerful. These include the special circumstances of promise making and taking, relationships between adults and children arising out of parenting, the vulnerable situation of the citizen accused of a crime, and, especially for our purposes, the special circumstances of the doctor-patient relationship. When a promisee accepts a promise, he or she has moral rights not also held by the promisor, specifically, the right to enforce or not enforce the promise. Were this not the case, promisees would be easily manipulated by promisors and the multiple human goods attained by the practice of promising would be lost. Children have special moral rights against their parents for proper upbringing, an upbringing designed to educate and liberate the person of the child and to bring him or her to competent and autonomous adulthood. Without these inarticulate but valid claims by children and parents' respect for them in general, children would be subject to extremes of exploitation. Accused criminals have special moral rights since persons held against their wills in official custody by others are highly subject to abuse. Patients have special moral rights against their physicians and other health care providers since without them their relative lack of medical knowledge and their pain and anxiety would make them vulnerable to all kinds of assaults on their lives and autonomies.

In all of these cases and in others like them, the recognition of special rights helps to restore the equality presumed by our ideal of the human person, an equality lost because of the far superior factual power of one member of the relationship. But again, these are not truly new nor additional rights, but a further factual specification of the same equal human rights had ideally by each and every human person. These special moral rights can work themselves into law as some of our examples indicate. This is appropriate since special rights take greater cognizance of the fact world

73

than do general moral rights, and it is in their dogged connection to that same fact world that legal rights have their peculiar moral value.

In ideal, then, we are all equally valuable persons with equal human rights. The recognition of these ideal rights has been and will continue to be factually incomplete as we work and hope for moral progress. At the same time, we do our ideals the honor of recognizing them in the concrete when we admit that general human rights must be made particular and unequal when special circumstances make real human relationships particular and dangerously unequal.

C. Beyond Duty

The ethical principle we have formulated, the maximization of practical personal autonomy, happiness, and pleasure within the bounds of respect for the rights of all persons, clearly urges us to go beyond duty. Duty as we have seen is inhibitory and conservative. It preserves in our personal and social habits the achievements of rights recognized in the past. The moral drive to attain value, on the other hand, is dynamic and constantly moves us toward new goods. When it is clear that the rights of all persons involved have not been compromised, our autonomy maximization principle urges us to maximize human satisfactions in moral consciousness, in mind, and in body. Thus, we seek for the greatest amount of factual awareness and exercise of each person's incalculable value as a center of value creative activity, and then the greatest amount of happiness and pleasure for all persons involved; all of this consistent with our duties to all persons.

What makes for human pleasure is relatively clear given the constancies of the human body. What makes for happiness is less clear but may be broadly determinable within a given culture at a given time. Certainly, the use of social statistics can indicate patterns of unhappiness in a society through the compilation of data on suicides, poverty, unemployment, drug addition and alcoholism, crime, warfare, and like expressions of human suffering. Such findings may at least provide a negative approach toward maximizing happiness by allowing us to seek to minimize these and other sources of suffering. What is least clear in our ethical principle is what can be done to enhance human autonomy, so we turn to that now.

Each individual human person is, on our account, an incalculably worthy center of value creative activity, the value of values. We have just emphasized the implications of this view for human equality: If we are all incalculably worthy, we are equal in worth. Yet the facts of the case differ considerably. In spite of the validity in ideal of our prior argument that every person is so worthy because the self of each person is the source of value for his or her own world of experience, in fact many persons do not see themselves or others in this light. The first task then of one who would maximize the attainment of practical personal autonomy is to promote the self-consciousness of this incalculably valuable autonomy in each in-

74

dividual person. Persons should develop a proper sense of self-esteem, a sense appropriate to the value we have ascribed to each of them. One obvious way to develop such self-esteem is through clarifying the situation of the self as the value source in a person's life. This can be done in the abstract and ideal as we have done here through philosophical reflection.

For most persons, however, this air is too thin. The great majority of persons depend day to day primarily on their emotions and habits rather than on their reasoning. We have seen that there are good reasons why this should be so. Admitting this, the conclusions of our rational discussions must be brought into persons' lives through their emotions and habits. This is especially imperative with children. They must be helped to feel their incalculable worth and to express that feeling as they build their habits. But what is true of children is generally true to some extent of adults as well, so that a similar if less dramatic point can be made about the need for adults to feel and express their worth in their daily habits. With children and with adults, this can be done only when the significant other persons in their lives recognize not only the radical equality of all persons, but also the radical uniqueness of each person, of this person. To treat two persons scrupulously the same without recognizing the special needs and talents of each may discharge one's duty but may do so in an unnecessarily value impoverished fashion. To give each of two children a guitar, for example, though one wanted a drum is to treat them equally but insensitively. To distribute all labor among adults equally though some are clearly talented in one way and others in another is to equalize mechanically and without a sense for the individuality of persons. Persons can feel their own self-worth in their actions only if the community of persons around them respects their individuality even as they respect their equality. In this way, the ideal self-esteem of persons can become clarified in fact.

This is no easy task as the tension between this discussion and the prior one on equality indicates. Acknowledging the unique needs of one person may appear to be arbitrary treatment from another person's point of view and thus a violation of this other person's rights. One must always remain sensitive to the possible validity in such objections. But this is the nature of the challenge of attaining new and important values even as we discharge our duties: Duty demands similarity but our values seek uniqueness. Perhaps the model of a harmonious family can shed some light on the kind of solution possible here. In such a family, children are treated differently because of age and special needs and talents. Achievement of a sense of family harmony demands that over time there must emerge a shared sense of fairness, a sense that though this child may get more attention now, the other children will get their proper share of attention as well, even if it expresses itself in different ways and at different times. This context of fairness creates an atmosphere of mutual trust within which exceptions to mechanically equal treatment are accepted as good for everyone over the long run. Carrying this model into adult relationships and into our social habits is difficult but the attempt is a worthy one. One must constantly be aware of the demands of duty but also of the need to discharge them in such a way that individual self-esteem is maximized and practical personal autonomy is enhanced. Our duty to persons derives from their radical equality of worth but that estimation of worth is ultimately grounded in the radical uniqueness of each person's self. Going beyond duty here means enhancing the factual awareness of that uniqueness in an overall scheme of equality.

In addition to the factual clarification of a person's self-worth, human autonomy can be enhanced by promoting among persons a sense of their concrete relatedness with other persons. Nothing builds a person's self-esteem more than close and emotively positive relationships with other persons. Mutual respect, friendship, and love between persons confirms each person's self-worth through the reflection of that worth in another's respect, concern, and affection. I think of myself as a more valuable person when I see that you value me too. Your very valuing of me increases my valuing of you as it increases my sense of self-value. The same can be said of you if our relationship is reciprocal. Thus, a mutually reinforcing valuing relationship can build between persons. At its minimal development, this relationship is one of mutual respect. At a deeper level, this is friendship. At the most profound level, this is love. Mutual respect, friendship, and love build self-esteem and an atmosphere of trust and concern within which each person can more freely and rationally exercise his or her own value creative activity. Persons in such positive relationships promote each other's self-transcending process of ideal realization.

It is also true that there are certain human dispositions which can make the building of such relationships easier or more difficult. Mutual respect, friendship, and love are made easy when persons are habituated toward tolerance of others' differences, toward attitudes of sharing in work and play, and toward feelings of empathy with the emotive and cognitive struggles of others. These same self-affirming human relationships are made more difficult, often impossible, when persons take on habits of dogmatic self-righteousness, selfishness in work and play, and indifference to the lot of others. Thus, the promotion of mutual respect, friendship, and love between persons and attainment of the important consequences these relationships have for personal self-esteem and practical personal autonomy depend on active inculcation of these positive habits among children and throughout adult relationships in society.

There is also a curious irony about human self-esteem as it bears on relations with others that must be noted here. It appears to be paradoxical but true that one of the most effective means of building personal self-esteem is through self-sacrifice for others. This self-sacrifice is not directly interested in enhanced self-esteem at all but is genuinely motivated by a true concern for others; paradoxically, enhanced self-esteem often emerges here even though it is not directly sought. It is commonplace for persons to claim that they found themselves and their true happiness in working for others. Not only saints and heroes, but also the most ordinary of men and women find considerable and profound self-worth in their multiple sacrifices for families, neighbors, friends, communities, churches, etc. Perhaps this insight lies at the heart of the continued vitality of Christianity: that selfless concern for others can be one of the most self-affirming of life attitudes.[11] In any case, the phenomenon of finding self-value through self-sacrifice is so prevalent and of such obvious value not only for the individual person, but also for the whole of society, that such a disposition ought to be inculcated among children and adults as well. This point also has a special bearing on our discussion of rights. If one has a right to claim something, one also has the right not to claim that something, the right not to exercise one's right. Both the common good and the autonomy maximization demanded by our ethical principle require the production of large numbers of persons who not only claim their due rights when appropriate, but who also "know" when it is best not to claim their rights; persons who "know" when the value concerns of others should be allowed to take temporary precedence over duties owed to them. Such a spirit of self-sacrifice helps to keep rights claims a serious and useful part of our moral discourse even as it serves, paradoxically, the autonomy interests of the very persons who so sacrifice a bit of themselves.

Finally, factually relevant advances in the enhancement of human autonomy can come through criticism at the personal and social levels. Since one's practical personal autonomy is shaped in fact by habit, one can develop real autonomy by criticizing one's habits in light of the standard of the self as the value of value. Do my habits bring me ever closer to the factual realization of this ideal or do they carry me further away and thwart my attainment of the ideal? Such self-criticism is an important part of all personal moral progress. If it is to be truly progressive, it must be constructive even at this introspective level. Brooding self-recrimination and fixation on one's faults can be as damaging to the enhancement of self-esteem as self-deluding egoism and bad faith denial of all fault. Constructive self-criticism must acknowledge the inevitablity of the gap between the ideal and the factual self. Growth in the right direction is the appropriate standard here.[12] One must ask not, "am I short of my ideal again?" but rather, "have I made any advance in the right direction, am I better today in some respect than I was yesterday?" This sort of constructive criticism can strengthen confidence in all of one's free and rational choosing, a confidence born out of a sense that the value creative activity of the self is growing in the right direction.

Criticism of the behavior of others is an even more sensitive task, as we all know from experience. Yet all persons, and especially children, need the resistance of the views of others to shape and fix their own views and so to grow in self-worth and the ability to freely and rationally choose for themselves. Reason must have a prior context of emotive presumption and active habit and this prior context can be shaped through continuous and constructive criticism of the actions of others. Here again, the standard must not be the ideal itself but progress toward the ideal. And as we all know, the criticism of others is seldom effective outside a context of mutual trust, a trust built through compliment of achievement as well as criticism of fault and through openness for criticism in return. As is becoming increasingly clear, the permissively raised child, that is, the child who grows without systematic and constructive criticism, becomes an unhappy adult with a poor sense of self-esteem and nagging doubts about the validity of his or her own autonomous choices.[13] Since our childhood shades ever so gradually into adulthood, a similar result is likely true for adults as well. Without constructive criticism in a context of mutual trust, adults too may become unhappy, low in self-esteem, and less practically autonomous.

There is no criticism so important, however, as criticism of the received social habits that form the horizon for the development of all persons within a given society. We have already seen that the ideal of the autonomous person which animates our concerns requires the companion ideal of a progressive society. Such a society can transcend itself because of its open institutionalized habits and the full participation of persons throughout its multiple practices and associations. On the other hand, when a society exhibits habits that lower personal self-esteem and practical personal autonomy, these habits must be brought to public attention and criticized in terms of the standards implied by the self as the value of value. If persons need factual clarification of their own worth and self-affirming relationships with others to do so, then society must have the institutionized structures to support such needs. First among these necessary social structures is political democracy based on the recognition of individual rights of liberty and access to needed goods and services and on equal access to governmental authority and office. Such political democracy sets the stage for the possibility of free, rational, and peaceful criticism and change of all other social institutions. Only with a foundation in political democracy can a society insure the possibility of its own self-transcendence and provide for the enhanced personal autonomy of all its citizens.

Political democracy can be regarded as the social expression of our duty to treat all persons equally. Our ethical drive to maximize attainment of all human values thus makes political democracy a conservative and inhibiting force within the larger meaning of democracy as a dynamic and progressive value. Democracy therefore is not only a political ideal for a progressive society, but an ideal which should pervade all social structures by way of the free and equal participation of persons in the institutions and practices that shape their lives. We are duty bound to share political governance equally; but autonomy maximization drives us to assert the value of democracy in all of our social habits. Nothing is so debilitating to the growth of practical personal autonomy than powerlessness over the events which factually control one's life, a sense of alienation and exclusion from the decision-making that affects one's future in the family, work place, school, church, neighborhood, economy, etc. All social habits must come increasingly under the control of this ideal of democratic participation in the powers and decision-makings that govern social life. In this manner, social mechanisms will be in place for the continued maximization of real human autonomy.

These considerations on the values that morally drive us above and beyond duty are admittedly sketchy and incomplete. Perhaps this will inevitably be so since the dynamism of value seeking is all consuming and the ideals of personal autonomy and progressive societies are inherently vague. Still, there is a real motivation here that takes us beyond the morally minimal in life and gives morality a texture, complexity, and potential for growth that commitment to duty alone cannot provide. Earnest appreciation of the incalculable value of each value creating self will inevitably propel us beyond the protection of human autonomy so far achieved to its active maximization in the future. Such a value drive will always bear the mark of human creativity.

III. Using the Tools: The Personal Core of Medical Care

Chapter 7.

The Sick Person

A. Sickness as Emergence of Body and Mind

We have now seen something of the ideals of autonomous persons in progressive societies and have explored several dimensions of morality and ethics. If it is true that morality as lived and ethics as reflection on that part of life are both ultimately shaped and animated by the ideals embedded within them, then morality and ethics, because of their direct relationship to human action, will be the tools with which persons try to more fully realize their ideals in fact. The proof of their usefulness as tools can only be found in their applications to concrete human situations and practices. Since our concern is contemporary medical care, we must now see if these tools of a morality and ethics focused explicitly on ideals are useful for the understanding and reshaping of concrete situations and practices in the medical care of persons. The ideals we have chosen are those of autonomous persons in progressive societies, ideals which are in most harmony with the nature of human reality as itself shaped by ideals and with the most progressive factual achievements of contemporary societies. Since these ideals center on the value of the person, it is appropriate that we begin the concrete use of our tools with a consideration of the subject of medical care: the sick human person. This beginning will help us to clarify the very purpose of medicine by helping to make explicit various elements of the sick world.

As we have already established, life as lived is experienced as a contextual unity. Reflective thought may attend to certain parts of this unitary experience and then extinguish itself into a renewed contextual whole, a whole enriched by latent experience of those parts. This is the mechanism by which we have uncovered the nature and value of the self. Attention to that part of our experience which is the source of our ability to value other persons, objects, and activities has allowed us to develop a reflective and positive self-consciousness. This positive self-consciousness may now, it is hoped, reenter and reshape the emotive and habit bound unity of experience as a personal and social enrichment, as a latent consciousness of oneself and others as incalculably valuable creators of value.

Not all self-consciousness is similarly benign. For example, finding oneself the only one in strange dress at what was announced as a costume party develops a self-consciousness too, but one that is embarrassed, uncomfortable, and belittling. In such a case, so long as the party lasts there is no return to the lived unity of normal experience. Instead, self-consciousness remains a burden, a continued negatively felt fragmentation of experience.

Such negative self-consciousness attaches to a common experience which one might call the emergence of the body. On most occasions, we are not directly aware of our bodies at all. They are transparent to us as we focus on the external world of other persons, objects, and activities. We live through our bodies with the ease and the naturalness of the whole moment we are experiencing and acting within.[1] Just as I do not normally think or say to myself "now I shall grasp for that door handle" but simply grasp for it; nor "now I will move this leg up to that step" but simply climb the stairs; in like manner, I do not normally think of my body as an instrument needing the explicit direction of my intentions. I simply move my body and do these actions spontaneously. Generally, the body is not something we are aware of as an aspect of our experience. It is wholly and unconsciously submerged within the contextual unity of experience. But there are times when consciousness directs itself to the body, times when the body emerges. Clearly, the experience of a pain is such a time, especially when I refer it to a specific area of my body. When my hand hurts, for instance, my hand emerges in my consciousness, fragments the otherwise unitary nature of my experience, and tends to dominate the moment. Such bodily emergence also occurs when I am trying to learn a new physical skill, like riding a bicycle or driving a car. In these cases I become bodily self-conscious since I direct many of my bodily movements with explicit intentions. This self-consciousness is heightened considerably when these explicit intentions are not spontaneously expressed in action because of lack of natural ability or acquired skill. In these cases, the body weighs on consciousness and appears to it as dull and inept, as the instrument that should spontaneously act but does not.

One can speak of the emergence of the mind in a parallel fashion. Ordinarily, we do not think of ourselves as having a mind as a piece or an aspect of our experience, since consciousness as it directs itself toward external persons, objects, and activities is also transparent to itself. We experience through our consciousness; we think through our minds. Seldom do we think of them. But there are times when a negative self-consciousness of one's mind can emerge. An emotional distress, for instance, often fixes my attention on my own consciousness, on my own mind that feels this bad feeling. Errors and mental incapacities of any sort also bring the mind before itself negatively. When I am correct about something, it is as if that correctness were part of the world itself; when I am mistaken, it is I alone who have been mistaken. In the experience of being correct, the mind sees the world and not itself, but in the experience of being mistaken, the world is momentarily lost as the mind focuses on itself as the source of error.[2] Such mental emergence also occurs when a cognitive endeavor becomes too demanding for my talents and skills. Here my consciousness is a weight on itself and appears dull, incompetent, and of little service.

A characteristic mark of the world of the sick person is this negative self-consciousness. This is not here due to low self-esteem. The sick person may, even when sick, have a higher self-esteem than many of the perfectly healthy. Instead, this negative self-consciousness is a function of the sort of emergence which fragments the normal unity of experience and refuses to be reabsorbed into a new unity so long as the individual remains sick. There may be persons who have diseases of considerable magnitude but who are not sick in this sense because the disease has not yet manifested itself in the emergence of body or mind. There may also be persons who have no demonstrable disease at all and yet who are clearly sick in this sense. Sickness here will mean this habit of fragmenting one's consciousness with a bad feeling about an emergent body or mind or both. This experience of destroyed or impaired unity is central to the misery of being sick. One's body, mind, or both just will not go away, and participation in one's normal range of activities is thus made difficult or impossible. This loss of one's normal activities seriously compromises one's practical personal autonomy by restricting its usual expressions.[3] Of course, sickness can be a matter of degree. It can vary in severity depending upon the strength of the negative emotion, the degree of the habit of fixating consciousness, the relative insistence of the emergent body, mind, or both, and the nature and number of normal activities made difficult or impossible.

Again, the most obvious case of sickness is physical pain. When sickness brings physical pain, it thoroughly and negatively commands and absorbs consciousness. One attends to its coming and going, to its degrees, to its spread to other parts of the body. Thus, the bodily instrument which we normally live through spontaneously becomes the conscious object of attention itself. And, of course, not only does pain so fixate consciousness, it also hurts. Indeed, it is because of its hurting and at times hurting badly, that pain can so dominate our attention and fragment the unity of consciousness. This fixation and hurting make the sick person unable or uninterested in pursuing his or her normal activities. Thus, in addition to the negative self-consciousness and the hurt, persons in pain are robbed of the autonomy, happiness, and pleasure which their normal activities can bring.

Mental sufferings affect us similarly. Emotional extremes, cognitive impairments, or both bring direct suffering in themselves. Our natural and social environment presents itself to us as affective through and through, from the spontaneous liking or antipathy for another person to the felt security of a familiar place, to the contentments and discontentments shot through our experience of our daily activities. Emotional imbalance distorts or removes this powerful and important affective texture. Such an imbalance pervades consciousness as one comes to habitually feel bad about one's feelings themselves. Knowledge or suspicion of impairment in cognitive skills can equally spread throughout consciousness as one begins to worry if decisions made and conclusions drawn are valid or functions of the impairment itself. Clear and adequate cognition is a central link between a person's internal life and the social world of others. Knowledge of cognitive impairment or suspicion of such impairment can withdraw a person from the social world and can lead to the sufferings of loneliness, alienation, and paranoia. This loss of psychological control and of the supportive emotional ambience in which it normally operates also destroys or diminishes one's real exercise of autonomy.[4]

There are other less obvious sources of negative self-consciousness when sick. Incapacity of any sort can become an insistent fragment of experience, a fragment which will not yield to a new unity of consciousness. Difficulties in moving the body as a whole or in its parts remind one of sickness at every turn and draw one away from activities which were previously enjoyed and were thus self-affirming. My not being able to do something, especially if it is something I once could do, can then lead directly to a negative self-consciousness in the other sense, that is, to a lowered sense of self-esteem. This lowered self-esteem, in light of a former, higher self-estimate, can itself be a powerful source of suffering for the sick.

Another feature of sickness which absorbs consciousness in this negative fashion is the dependence on others which it often involves. Even though we are all dependent on others in many profound ways when we are healthy, the peculiar dependence of the sick appears as a direct loss of practical personal autonomy and especially as a loss of freedom. The thought of losing rational control over important decisions in life is a significant cause of the suffering of the sick. Few adults view the prospect of a return to the docility of childhood and the consequent reliance on the proxy consent of others with anything but dread. Responsible exercise of autonomy may often be a burden, but it is one we are extremely reluctant to put down. In our society, independence and freedom are so highly valued that the dependencies and captivity of sickness are causes of suffering themselves. Finally, the sick can become negatively obsessed with their dependence on others by the thought of the cost of such dependence. The financial costs of a stay in a contemporary hospital, for example, can be so staggering that contemplation of one's bill and its impact on personal or familial budgets can itself bring suffering. Even where family or friends provide the needed help themselves without the aid of professionals, the sense of being a burden on others and the thought of the freedoms and normal activities this care is costing those helpful others can prey on one's mind. A not infrequent lament of the sick is pertinent here: "I can cope with the disease, but I hate being a burden on others."

Finally, a significant source of the habitual negative self-consciousness in sickness is the fact that dysfunctions of the body or mind are symbolic of our ultimate personal destinies: decline and death. A mere toothache can provoke the image of toothless old age. A pain in the lung can bring a foreboding of cancer. A forgotten memory can portend senility. Thus, mental and physical sickness can breed a more profound kind of sickness, a fixation on our inevitable deterioration. There is no escaping the fact that after we reach adulthood, many of our bodily functions are in decline; this is palpable by middle age. A wound slow to heal, the finger that no longer moves properly, the new pains found in exercises which used to delight; these can become reminders of the impermanence and wearing down of the body. And they can negatively fixate consciousness. Serious injuries or losses of function can directly intimate death. Fear of dying and anxiety about what may lie beyond is never far from the consciousness of one seriously sick. The negative character of fixation on this great imponderability of all human life is made that much worse in a society which glorifies youth and health and which denies the fact of personal mortality so far as and whenever it is able.[5] The possible connection of any sickness with this ultimate contingency of our existence is sufficient cause in itself for generating a negative and absorbing self-consciousness of body and mind.

For these reasons, and for the consequent loss or diminishment of practical personal autonomy which it causes, sickness is an evil in human life. There is the possibility, as with any evil, that good may come of it. Enriched self-understanding, closer relationships with family and friends, a deeper spirituality, even the acts of care and concern by others which sickness generally provokes; all of these and many other goods may come from sickness. But in itself, sickness is a significant source of human misery. Our moral traditions, the ethical principle we have elaborated here, and the historical commitment of medicine compel us to seek to minimize this suffering and to eliminate or prevent it where possible.

B. Wellness as Wholeness

Except for the malingerer, persons who are sick seek to leave that state as quickly and as completely as possible. This is to say the obvious, since sickness involves pain, suffering, and loss of autonomy through the fixated, negative self-consciousness we have described. Sickness is an evil and we are normally and naturally repelled by it. But what is the state we wish to attain when we are sick? The answer to this question is critical since it will bear directly on the goals of medicine. Surely we want not to be sick, but what do we want to achieve? The most immediately plausible answer is health. When we are sick, we want to return to health; we want to be healthy again.

As intially plausible as this appears, there are significant problems in defining the notion of health in a manner clear enough for it to be both accurate to our common experience of being free of sickness and useful as a practical goal for the care of sick persons. To show why this is so, we can begin by considering one of the most ideal and comprehensive definitions of health put forward in recent years, that of the World Health Organization.[6] According to W.H.O., health is "complete physical, mental, and social well-being and not merely the absence of disease or infirmity." While this may be a suitable ideal definition of health, for a variety of reasons it is not sufficiently practical, that is, it is not an ideal we are capable of attempting to realize in fact.

In the first case, the inclusion of social well-being in this definition clearly must signal an analogous use of the term 'health.' Surely social well-being is not suggested by the ordinary use of the term, except when we are conscious of using it in a wider and thus analogous sense, as when we judge a whole society to be healthy or sick. At times, we do assert that a whole society was sick, the late period of the Roman empire, or example. But we are conscious here that this is an analogy, a metaphor.[7] Just as a dying person generally faces decline, loss of integrated physical and cognitive functions, confusion in will, etc.; so the historian can isolate social factors in Rome in the third and fourth centuries which appear to express similar phenomena at the collective level. But this social decline, disintegration, and loss of will is at best analogous to the root meaning of the term, the use we mean when we say it of individual persons. It is true as well that we speak of certain social relationships as being healthy or unhealthy. For example, one might judge as unhealthy a romantic relationship in which both parties reinforce each other's worst habits, as in the case of one's submissiveness fostering further the other's tendency to dominate and vice versa. By contrast, social relationships that draw out latent talents, generate new interests, and tend to balance a personality; such relationships we often describe as healthy ones. Nevertheless, in all of these cases, the use of 'health' is an extension from its core use, an analogy or a metaphor. As such, the inclusion of this social element, while it does respond to some important dimensions of human life, obscures rather than clarifies what we mean by 'health.' Certainly a sick person's immediate goal is not clarified at all by reference to social well-being.

There is a further, more onerous implication in the notion of social well-being. If the meaning of 'health' is extended by implication to the whole of society, then we are led to suppose that there may be doctors or similar experts to whom one can go to maintain or restore health for all of society. But who are these doctors, these social experts? Surely every society will have those who can offer expert opinions on social questions, but politically democratic societies can not allow experts to choose and act on these opinions in the manner in which a doctor often chooses and acts for his or her patients. The alleged existence of experts for the cure of sick societies is the basis on which many authoritarian and totalitarian societies have claimed legitimacy. If a society is truly sick and some elite claims to have the cure for this social sickness, there is a strong temptation for the elite to bypass consent of the persons governed and to base their authority on direct appeal to the social need for therapy directed toward a return to health. Though justifications like this can be found in most authoritarian and totalitarian societies, there is a particularly graphic expression of it today in the Soviet Union where political dissent is regarded as a sickness treatable by psychiatry.[8] Such a punitive and abusive use of psychiatry debases both the politics of that society and medicine itself. Since the introduction of alleged medical experts on social issues is so dangerous to political democracies, and since it relies on what appears to be a metaphor, this element of the W.H.O. definition is best omitted altogether. If the political realm is an arena for free and rational public debate and decision as political democracy would have it, then the general moral words of 'good' and 'bad', 'right' and 'wrong' are more appropriately said of a society than 'healthy' and 'sick.'

One might also wonder whether **complete** physical and mental well-being is something that human beings are even capable of. There are few days even in the healthiest of lives in which some physical malady does not express itself. Would the existence, for instance, of headaches, indigestion, or occasional insomnia remove one from the category of the healthy? Further, the idea of **complete** mental well-being is likely an empty notion itself if the presumption of Freudian psychology is correct that each of us has some mental illness, at least some neurosis which we live with and accept as relatively normal. Would the existence of anxiety, guilt, and fear remove one from the category of the healthy? Freud aside, anxiety and guilt seem to be too much a part of all human choice to be considered unhealthy in themselves. And what of the reasonable fears in our mental life: of crime, of war, of death, of nuclear annihilation? Do these fears make us all unhealthy?

Furthermore, even if we were to pare down this ambitious definition to read that health is the absence of disease or infirmity, problems remain. There are significant cultural differences in what counts as a disease in a given society at a given time.[9] Contemporary Americans regard tooth decay and gum diseases as unhealthy, for example, yet most persons the world over and throughout history have accepted the loss of teeth in middle and old age with the same inevitability with which we approach male hair loss. Were all of these persons unhealthy even when they did not know it? In more general terms, what does the absence of disease really mean? If it means absence of disease symptoms, there will be those who are subjectively healthy on this account but who have objective diseases that are as yet asymptomatic, early stages of cancer for example. On the other hand, if absence of disease means objective absence of the disease itself regardless of symptoms, many persons who appear to themselves and to others to be the "picture of health" will be factually unhealthy.

This last suggestion, the definition of health as the objective absence of disease favors the scientific dimension of contemporary medicine. A physician reading an X-ray knows that the person across the desk is unhealthy regardless of how that person subjectively feels or what others may think. The nurse reading the charts and vital signs of a patient may know that that patient is not getting any healthier regardless of what he or she may subjectively perceive. And we can objectively define gum disease in dental science regardless of what a given culture may perceive. These cases suggest that health may be a natural and objective norm whose presence or absence is determinable by a properly trained, i.e. scientifically trained, professional.

But the subjective dimension of a person's feelings and thoughts about health are far too important to eliminate from any acceptable definition of health. The cultural perception of sickness and health controls the responses of persons in that society to conditions of the body and mind. If a culture holds that this condition is a sickness, the normal activities of the person with that condition change or cease, and when a culture holds that this condition is not a sickness, those same activities go on unchanged. This impact of culture is too large to ignore since it regulates the formation of the negative self-consciousness we have described as the core of sickness. Thus, society shapes persons' abilities to maintain or lose practical personal autonomy in their normal activities. Also, we are becoming more and more aware of the power, in individual cases, of the placebo effect and its reverse, the power to literally make oneself more objectively healthy by the development of a positive subjective state and the power to literally make oneself more objectively unhealthy by the development of a negative subjective state.[10] Surely this does not account for all or even a great portion of health and disease, but it is such a graphic phenomenon when it occurs that the subjectivity of the person just cannot be ignored in any adequate definition of health.

Perhaps we can find a more adequate notion of health by taking a clue from our human perspective on health and disease in the plant and animal world. In general, we have a quite lofty view of the diseases of plants and animals. Since the causes and processes of any disease, whether in plant, animal, or human, follow the laws and courses of nature, diseases are quite natural in a straightforward way, every bit as natural as health itself. Though we may sense a loss, and at times an extreme loss, when these disease mechanisms take away a pet or some livestock, or when they destroy a flower garden or blight a crop; in general we regard the diseases and deaths of animals and plants as quite ordinary and nearly value free. Yet when these diseases and deaths do touch us emotionally or financially, we suspend our usual indifference, take them up into our value world, and lament them as sad or even disastrous.[11] A similar situation may prevail in our own case. Diseases which are objectively there in our bodies and minds may mean little or nothing to us until we take them up into our value world and read their implication as sad or disastrous. Minor tooth decay, a heart murmur, even hypertension and occasional mental depression can mean little or nothing to us as persons unless and until we consciously take them into our world of values. This taking of a disease in our value world can occur in multiple ways from the objective worsening of the condition and the consequent appearance of subjective symptoms to the condition being called to our subjective attention through some objective medical test.

This movement from indifference to concern suggests that the value creative activity of the self is critically involved. It is the value creative concern of the self which propels the sick person toward health. Using this insight, let us begin to define health as a valued sense of personal wellness, where wellness itself will mean the opposite of sickness. If sickness is the self-conscious and negative fixation on an emergent body or mind, then health as wellness is the restored contextual unity of experience in which the body or mind submerges again in consciousness. Consciousness in the well person again lives through the body and mind and does not fixate on either. It goes out to its normal activities without the divided or thwarted attention of a fragmented experience. Regaining health means that the negative self-consciousness of sickness is dissolved into the lack of self-consciousness of wellness. Health as wellness, then, is a return to wholeness. Health is the wholeness of a consciousness that is one with its experiences and actions. Of course, this contextual unity is episodically broken by conscious thought on a recurring basis but, as we have seen, such normal thought extinguishes itself back again into a renewed and part enriched wholeness. Thus, the self-consciousness of thought is compatible with, indeed is a natural expression of, wellness; whereas the negative self-consciousness of sickness is not, because it refuses to be reintegrated into the unconscious unity of experience. In wellness, the body and mind are transparent as we pursue our normal activities. In sickness, they stand in our way. When wellness gives us access once again to our normal activities, practical personal autonomy is restored as well. We can freely and rationally choose for ourselves once more. Of course, both of these states of wellness and sickness can be and usually are matters of degree; seldom are we wholly well or wholly sick. Nevertheless, even as a matter of degree, wellness as the restored or increased unity and autonomy of experience is the goal of the sick person and therefore of medicine itself.

Notice that this definition of health as wellness, while founded on the self's consciousness, is not entirely subjective. One cannot reasonably deny conscious attention to objectively bad health news by insisting on one's subjective good feelings. The news that one has cancer, for example, will itself begin the process of negative self-conscious fixation characteristic of sickness, and wellness will have been lost to that extent simply on the subjective weight of the objective report itself. One could say, paradoxically of course, that the person was well, though cancerous, before the news. This paradox may be increasingly forced on us by the growing diagnostic power of modern medicine. More and more, the objective news of bad health will itself begin the process of sickness as the self takes this bad news into its value world and develops a habit of feeling bad in its attending to the now emerged body and mind.

Central to this definition of health as wellness is the ability of the well person to participate in normal daily activities without nagging attention to the bodily or mental aspect of experience. But this means a maintenance or restoration of good feelings, old habits, and the practical autonomy of one's free and rational choices. In its most profound sense then, wellness is the physical and mental precondition for practical personal autonomy. It is the maintenance and restoration of this critical precondition of personal autonomy that medicine must take as its goal. Maintaining and restoring health understood as wellness can be a fit ideal for medical practice since it can be factually realized in part in most cases. With such a concept, medicine can have a goal which is clear, relevant to our experience, and practical; a goal meaningfully related to our ideals of autonomous persons in progressive societies.

C. The Plight of the Sick

In addition to the individual person's experiences of fragmentation of unity, there are also many significant social dimensions to sickness and wellness. Certain occupations, diets, and life-styles are highly correlated with the onset of certain sicknesses and these factors are expressions of the culture and the institutionalized habits of an entire society. The rates of black lung disease, coronary disease, and venereal disease, for example, are direct expressions of a society which burns and therefore mines coal, which consumes a great deal of fatty meats, and whose permissive ethos encourages multiple sexual contacts. Society, as has been suggested, even influences which of the objective conditions in nature will be regarded culturally as a disease. Since regarding a condition as a disease is a necessary part of producing sickness, our societies influence our very having of sicknesses.

At the same time, societies, through their institutions and practices, structure ways of getting and staying well. Attempting to stay well in one society may dictate diet and exercise programs; in another, religious ritual. Restoring health in one society may mean seeking a university trained physician; in another, a traditional herbalist or shaman. In one society, such health services may be paid for individually; in another, wholly or partly free. And since societies shape our perceptions of sickness, they will shape our perceptions of wellness too. Clearly we learn from our societies patterns of fixing negatively on the body or mind and patterns of living through these same bodies and mind without conscious attention.

Also, the sick take on certain social roles in society. In our society, for example, the mentally sick are made into pariahs who are hidden in institutions; in other societies, they have been regarded with awe as special conduits for the spirit world. In our society, much attention has been paid to defining the sick role.[12] Since sickness is largely thought to be something that happens to us beyond our control, the sick are usually considered innocent victims of fate. They have a sickness they did not want and could not help from getting. Because of this, they are expected to want to get better, to return to wellness. This, in turn, entails the expectation that the sick will seek appropriate professional help to care for or cure sickness. When one gets sick beyond one's control, wants to get better, and seeks appropriate professional help to do so; when such conditions prevail, the most socially powerful dimension of the sick role comes into play: The sick are exempted from their usual daily responsibilities. This exemption is institutionalized in such various ways as sick days with pay and leaves for extended illness, and it shows itself in such practices as allowing sick children absences from school and tolerating the incivilities of co-workers with colds.

One might conceive of this exemption as a special right of the sick. Normally, our presumption of equality binds us all equally to daily obligations. The special circumstances of the sick, (pain, suffering, loss of autonomy through negative self-consciousness) lead us to acknowledge special rights for them because these circumstances make the sick highly vulnerable. Of course, there are other compelling practical reasons for such exemptions as well. Often, the sick literally cannot perform their normal duties. Often they get sicker when they try. Often they spread their sicknesses to others in their normal routine; and even when the disease is not spread itself, the negative self-consciousness of sickness sometimes is. But over and above these practical considerations, the sick role exemption is expressive of our intuitive and deeply felt sympathy for the sick. This habitual sympathy is the emotional force behind the exemption of the sick from their normal obligations.

Part of the plight of the sick in contemporary American society is that the sick role is undergoing considerable change, change which tends to make us less willing or less able to so exempt the sick. Unless we consciously attend to this change and work to mitigate its negative impact, the intuitive sympathy we now have for the sick may become lessened or lost and the predicament of the sick will be made that much worse because of our unreflective social habits. Let us, therefore, examine some of the factors that have begun to cause this change in the sick role.

In the first place, as we are becoming more and more aware of the part which occupation, diet, and lifestyle play in the making of sickness and wellness, there is an increasing tendency to see the sick no longer as helpless victims but as contributors to their sicknesses. A lifetime of highly compensated work in a chemical industry may trigger some terrible disease but knowing the hazards of such a profession, as we now do, is it not easier for us to think, if not to say, that such a person freely assumed these risks and was adequately compensated for them throughout his or her working life? Knowing now that too much fat in foods and too much alcohol can lead to heart disease, are we not less likely to feel that this overweight and heavy drinking coronary patient is wholly a victim of forces beyond his or her control? Knowing now that long time cigarette smoking causes lung cancer, under any reasonable interpretation of causation, are we not more likely to blame the lifelong cigarette smoker who now has cancer?[13] This point can, of course, be carried throughout the full range of sicknesses now known to be connected in some degree to human choice and habit. Even one's place of residence in a city or region has statistically demonstrable health implications. Are we not now more prone to feel that "she knew people in that area get a lot of pollution, what did she expect." Thus our dramatic increase in knowledge here has also increased our tendency to blame the victims of disease and sickness.

When we blame the sick for their sicknesses, we feel little sympathy for them, are reluctant to exempt them from their normal duties, and tend to make their negative self-consciousness all the more acute.

Secondly, we are not always sure any longer that every sick person wants to get better. There is a growing awareness of the problem of malingering, of the use of hospital beds by persons who have no demonstrable disease but who want to be considered sick for the exemption of the sick role, for the public and third party support involved, and for the attention and sympathy they may then get from others.[14] Persons suffering from long-standing abuse of alcohol and drugs often make repeat visits to emergency rooms with such frequency that one must wonder if they truly want to get well. Our expanded academic and medical sensitivity to mental illness has also created whole classes of persons whose dependence on psychiatric care is so long term that doubts arise in the public mind regarding their desire to be well.[15] All of the points made above about the connection between habit and sickness are relevant here too: If these habits are not changed, how sincerely does this person want to get well?

There are also new problems in the seeking of appropriate help when sick. Medical science and the development of multiple medical specializations, while they contribute to very high quality care, also create an extreme fragmentation in medicine. In many cases, it is hard for the lay person to know what medical help is needed and available and how to go about securing it.[16] For example, the existential press of sickness generally makes the sick person a poor consumer. When looking for other important and expensive services in an economy such as ours, the smart consumer takes his or her time. This consumer reads service information, seeks advise from friends and relatives, and shops for the best quality at the best price. Securing the appropriate medical help does not fit this market model. A person who is sick, especially one who is very sick, or suspects that he or she may be cannot and should not take his or her time. There are few publicly available and frank sources of information concerning medical services; advice from friends and relatives by and large is spotty and anecdotal in character; appraising the quality of medical services generally and that of particular physicians and hospitals is notoriously difficult; and shopping for the lowest price is out of the question when life or a significant health question is at stake. If I need a competent brain surgeon and I need one fast, who do I ask for direction; how do I know such direction is reliable if I get it; will I be able to check on quality; and will I even bother to check on price?

The publicity given to alternative therapies at the edges of medical research has also promoted confusions in seeking appropriate help. Should a late stage cancer patient accept the latest experimental drug from contemporary scientific medicine though little hope is offered for its success or should he or she try a nontraditional drug or dietary approach? The media, the medical and anti-medical literature, and the experiences of friends and relatives abound with confusions here.

All of these factors conspire to mitigate the spontaneous exemption we would otherwise extend to the sick and tend to sap our reservoir of sympathy for them. What exemptions do we feel inclined to extend toward the chronically overweight person who never exercises and who now takes his back pain to a chiropractor? What sympathy do we feel for the lifelong cigarette smoker whose late stage lung cancer has driven her to another country for a "cure" ridiculed by establishment medicine? How do we regard the person whose ignorance of where and how to get appropriate medical care has worsened his previously curable condition to the point of incurability? These changes in our social habits are placing great pressure on the sick role and our attitudes towards those who assume it. Again, it is pertinent to point out that the social horizon against which this is occurring is that of a society that glorifies youth and health and denies or disguises sickness, old age, and death.

If we are to mitigate this increasing social burden of those who are already suffering personally from their sicknesses, we shall have to adopt some conscious strategies in line with our ideals of autonomous persons in progressive societies and our ethical principle of maximizing practical personal autonomy. Three such strategies suggest themselves.

First, even as we work to promote personal and social habits that will make for the prevention of sickness and the promotion of wellness, we must not blame the victims of life-style related diseases. In no individual case can science or medicine determine which were the most critical determining factors and which factors were only supporting. Many people smoke cigarettes and never develop lung cancer, for example. Some smoke very little and do. Clearly then, in addition to personal habit there are other factors at work even in the obvious life-style related diseases. In all likelihood, chief among these other factors is a genetically determined susceptibility for which no person can rightfully be blamed. I did not ask for or merit the body whose constitution may make me less resistant to cancer nor did you ask for or merit your constitution which may make you more resistant. More importantly, as none of us has access to the internal life of others, none of us knows directly of the strengths and weaknesses of the will that has shaped the habit in question. Perhaps the habit of cigarette smoking of this sixty year old man was begun by his insecure and peer conscious teenage self, and by the time his adult self desired to stop smoking the habit was already too well fixed. Perhaps this heavy drinker has tried to stop and tried earnestly on any number of occasions; maybe she has put more conscious effort, albeit without result, into maintaining her health than a multitude of others who by chance or genetics never found drinking attractive at all and therefore have never had to try to stop.

These perspectives are not expressive of a retreat from personal autonomy. In the ideal, all of us are free and rational agents. But the accidents of genetic disposition, psychological makeup, and the ubiquitous human phenomenon of weakness of the will often drive ideally autonomous persons to factual habits of which they are truly victims.

Respect for the incalculable value of each person, regardless of his or her habits, should lead us to systematically suspend the assignment of responsibility and blame to sufferers of life-style related diseases. One last speculative remark is appropriate on this point: chances are very good that one day nearly all sickness will be scientifically related to some life-style choices and habits. Since we will all become sick and we all have life-styles and habits, the "Golden Rule" insight is applicable here. We should build habits of extending to sick others, regardless of life-style, the same sympathy we would want in similar circumstances for ourselves.

Secondly, we must guarantee to all persons quick and sure access to quality medical care. A progressive society must institutionalize this access in some manner. If we genuinely bind ourselves to the value of the person, nothing can be a clearer social implication of that value than the need to provide social structures to save lives in emergency cases and to provide for the minimizing of sickness and the maximization of wellness in all cases.[17] Such social structures may take many forms consistent with other social values, but they will surely be inadequate if persons are effectively denied access to quality medical care because they did not know how to get it, what to get, or could not pay for it. If commitment to this ideal means practically that governments must create bureaucracies for the distribution and payment of health care, so be it. Bureaucracy is merely another name for politically sanctioned social habit and we are morally obliged to build social habits in line with our duties to others. The obligation to provide some level of quality medical care equally available to all is too palpably a part of what it means to maximize practical personal autonomy and to respect the incalculable value of each human person to be denied.

Finally, part of the frenzy which attaches to the search for non-traditonal "cures" in the last stages of terminal diseases expresses a misapprehension on the part of the public and to some extent on the part of medicine itself, a misapprehension of medicine's primary goal. The goal of medicine cannot be cure in all cases. Each of us will ultimately be failed by medical cures regardless of how powerful they may become, because each of us is a mortal human being. While we work and should work to cure as many diseases as possible to lift the burden of sickness from humanity, we must be clear on this score. The primary goal of medicine is care and not cure. Cures we may sometimes provide, but care we must always provide. This is the most important special right of the sick — the right to be cared for, not only when cure is available but also when it is not. Restoring and insisting on the primacy of care over cure will itself go a long way to preserving and deepening our sympathy for the sick and for their increasingly difficult social role. Such a focus will also help to make it more likely that the autonomy of the sick human person is respected in the medical context.

Chapter 8.

The Health Care Professional and the Patient

A. Professionals in a Complex Society

It is a bromide but true that we live in a complex society. The twentieth century has witnessed some of the most significant advances in human knowledge and power since the beginnings of our species. Science has become a clear instrumentality for technology, and technology has changed the face of our planet and profoundly adjusted human relationships. From nuclear power to the telephone, from routine air travel to radio and television, ours has been a century of dramatic and ever accelerating change. Not all of this change has been for the better, of course. For the first time ever, we can entirely destroy our species and severely damage our planet with only a few reckless acts by only a few individuals. Telephones, radio, and television have had a negative effect on personal growth and self-education in many cases and in many ways. The list of like dangers and drawbacks is long and grows longer daily. Still, there are massive goods in our new knowledge and powers, goods which, if harnessed to the right ideals with the commitments of a sufficient number of strong and sincere wills, could significantly enhance the lives of persons and societies.

The ideals we have embraced and elaborated call for the use of this new knowledge and power in the service of producing autonomous persons in progressive societies. The fact is, however, that the growing complexity of our society makes it harder and harder for a single person to be truly autonomous. Daily, we are individually shaped and directed by the decisions of others, often nameless and faceless others; persons who make wars and peace, invent new machines for work and play, run our transportation and media. As the complexity and interdependence of our society grows, so does the individual's sense of being overwhelmed by events out of control. Even the most modest of contemporary households, for example, requires periodic attention by multiple experts because no one person can be a competent carpenter, plumber, electrician, TV repairman, etc. As our lives have become more complex, so our dependencies on expert service and advice has increased. Thus, an increase of the knowledge and power of our species has really meant a direct increase of knowledge and power for some persons in some situations and only indirectly through them for others.

Chief among the necessary experts in contemporary American society is the professional. In some of the most critical of life's moments, the average person does not have the requisite knowledge and power to make successful choices in his or her own best interest. The complexities of the law, for example, are too intricate and too weighty in consequence for the untrained individual and so the service of a lawyer is generally sought when a serious legal issue is at hand. In medicine, this is obviously the case. Except for the most trivial of conditions, the sick person must seek the assistance of the health care professional, doctors, nurses, dentists, pharmacists, etc. Thus, persons in general have become dependent on the professional expertise of the few.

This dependence on the knowledge and power of the professional in contemporary society creates a whole series of highly structured human relationships of marked inequality. The professional often has the lives and destinies of the client or patient in his or her hands, in the case of medicine often literally so. As we have seen, when relationships of inequality occur in such a systematic and highly structured fashion and around issues of such importance, special rights arise for the protection of the vulnerabilities of the dependent party. Consequent on the existence of these special rights are special duties on the part of the professional. Thus, a fiduciary relationship is formed in which the professional is duty bound as a professional to serve the best interest of the client or patient; and the client or patient has a special right to receive such fiduciary agency.

This is not to deny the fact that the professional also serves his or her own interests. Clearly, the contemporary professional is well compensated financially for services rendered; indeed, by contrast with similar education and effort in other fields and by comparison with standard compensations in their own recent pasts, contemporary professionals are often grossly overcompensated.[1] And, of course, the professional serves his or her own interests by the satisfactions derived from providing effective service directly to other persons who need and respect the professional's skills. The point, however, is that the very nature of being a professional binds one to the service of client or patient.[2] The personal interests of lawyers and doctors are served, too, but it is the interests of the persons served by them that must dominate their attention and motivate their choices and actions. As a whole person, the professional has as many value interests and duties as any other person in society including drives to make money, enhance reputation, find pleasure and happiness, etc. But considered only through that aspect of his or her life which is professional, the lawyer, physician, or other professional is obliged to suspend other value interests and duties so as to fix directly and exclusively on service to the interests of client or patient. Only in this manner can a progressive society insure institutions and practices through which persons overwhelmed by the complexities of events can return a measure of factually relevant autonomy to their lives. The professional in a complex society is a fiduciary agent for the maintenance and restoration of practical personal autonomy in the lives of the nonprofessionals whose interests are served.

Since our concern here is with medicine and since the context of medical care is usually under the authority of the physician, let us explore the special duties of the contemporary physician. The first and most compelling of the duties of physicians is to set in principle and regularly achieve in practice a high standard of care for patients.[3] Part of this duty is clearly collective; physicians as a group must evolve standards of professional practice and systematically bind individual physicians to those standards. It is part of the meaning of being a profession that society has granted it, in a legally binding fashion, special privileges, especially the privilege of a great measure of professional autonomy. Physicians have, for example, a legally enforced monopoly of practice since no citizen can advertise and perform medical services without recognized medical credentials. Thus, professionals are assured a certain range of freedom from the normal competitions of a market based economy. They are also given a wide ranging ability to make informed choices about what constitutes proper professional care, since the law routinely defers to the standards of the medical community in adjudicated legal conflicts involving medical care. For these reasons and for their own obvious self-interest, physicians through their professional organizations and through various peer review mechanisms at the local level must set the highest of standards for medical practice and enforce them throughout their profession. In a rapidly expanding field such as medicine, these standards cannot be fixed once and for all times. Instead, like our selection of ethical ideals, physicians must make free and reasonable choices of the best available standards. But unlike our selection of ideals, these standards should not set out vague desiderata but concrete descriptions of mandatory behavior. Once these standards are set, they must constitute effective boundaries for minimally acceptable professional behavior. Of course, the policing of these standards will be difficult since of necessity it will involve the criticism and penalizing of professional colleagues, of those whose practice falls below the minimum acceptable level. But this is a burden which the medical community must accept if it is to foster the maximization of practical personal autonomy among its patients and if it is to maintain the social trust necessary for its effective functioning. If the medical profession does not effectively police itself, then surely society will through its legislative organs. Then some of the important social autonomy of the medical professional will have been lost.

The individual physician in his or her practice is personally bound to these same standards of care. This entails that the individual physician must make every effort to understand the prevailing standards and to develop fixed habits of meeting and even surpassing them. One of the most important dimensions of physicians' standards of care, and one which has been recognized throughout the history of western medical practice, is the duty to avoid harming patients. **"Primum, non nocere"** or "first, do no harm" has long been recognized as one of the central moral elements of proper professional care for patients.[4] This choice for the priority of avoidance of harm over the doing of good represents in medical tradition the very same conclusion we have already drawn about ethics in general: Discharge your duties before increasing the attainments of value; avoid evil first, then do good. Clearly, patients seek medical care because they strongly desire to move from sickness to wellness. They have an insistent drive to secure the good of wellness and avoid the evil of sickness. In recognition of the compelling character of this desire on the part of patients and the extremes to which they will sometimes go to satisfy it, and recognizing as well patients' general vulnerability before the knowledge and skill of physicians, our medical tradition has insisted that physicians not harm patients, that they not do anything to make patients worse off than when they first sought professional assistance. Of course, many patients become worse off in spite of a physician's best efforts, but if that physician has exercised appropriate standards of care this inevitability is no violation of the **primum**. And of course, many modern medical techniques immediately harm a patient; the pain of an injection, the loss of an amputation, the many sufferings of chemotherapy, these and other procedures are clearly harms in themselves. But in the larger therapeutic context, these are usually not purely harms but harming aspects of what is overall a good, a cure, a release from pain, a prevention of future disease, an extension of life, etc. The harms which the **primum** forbids are direct and pure harms to patients, harms like negligence in advice or procedures, invasive and nonconsensual touching of a patient, using a patient experimentally to advance one's career or to make money, inflicting unnecessary surgeries and drug regimens, abandoning a patient in need, and violating confidences arising out of the doctor-patient relationship. There will, of course, be many times when a doctor can do little to actually help a patient, but in all cases commitment to professional standards of care requires that he or she at least refrain from inflicting these and similar harms on patients.

From the patient's perspective, the central special right is to this professional standard of care bounded by the **primum non nocere** principle, but other rights arise as well due to the patient's special needs. Furthermore, if we are to enhance practical personal autonomy as our ideals indicate, we will be driven to claim certain values for patients beyond mere recognition of their rights. A first consideration here involves the affective and habit bound nature of the patient's reliance on the professional's care. Though no one can guarantee a right to a cure, since a cure may not exist for the malady at hand or may not be efficacious in this particular case, patients have a right as persons to concerned and continuous care from their physicians. There is a clear and at times profound emotional dimension to sickness, a dimension consequent on the pain, suffering, loss of autonomy, and negative self-consciousness of sickness itself. This depth of feeling is brought into and becomes a large part of the therapeutic relationship from the patient's point of view. It is too much, perhaps impossible, to demand as a duty that physicians develop a warm and responsive emotive relationship with every patient, since physicians, like all of us, have their spontaneous likes and dislikes and many patients are not factually likeable by any standard. Still it is not too much to assert that maximization of the patient's value interests gives him or her a claim on the affective concern of their physicians. This concern need not be maudlin nor sentimental and it need not in principle take any more time than a doctor-patient exchange without such concern. A genuine feeling of concern can be clear-eyed and straightforward and can be conveyed in a moment by a joke, a gesture, a tone of voice. Demonstration of such human feeling is an important part of the affective dimension of healing and of patient satisfaction.[5] Patients, therefore, have a claim on such feelings if we would speed their healing and increase their satisfaction and thus maximize the restoration of their normal full range of pleasure, happiness, and practical personal autonomy.

Futhermore, patients have a right to continuous care. Patients habitually rely on the availability of their physician, a habit of reliance which can be dangerous if it is not routinely justified in fact. Once a doctor-patient relationship has been initiated and accepted by both parties, the doctor may not rightfully cease care unless the patient terminates the relationship, the therapy concludes by its own nature, there is mutual consent to terminate the relationship, or the doctor informs the patient of his intent to terminate care sufficiently in advance of termination to allow the patient to secure another doctor.[6] No doctor is duty bound to accept any given patient and, as the last condition for termination of the therapeutic relationship indicates, doctors may, after sufficient notice, reject any patient. Significant personal and social values may be secured, however, if doctors routinely go beyond duty to serve as wide a range of patients as possible, terminating therapeutic relationships only in the most intractable of cases.

Finally, our ideal of the autonomous person entails that patients have a right to a certain level of factual autonomy and an interest in as much more as is possible in their circumstances. Specifically, patients have a right to give or withhold informed consent over all aspects of their care.[7] Patients have a right to know what is being or will be done to them and why. Patients must be told the attendant risks of these proposed actions compared to alternative courses of action, including the alternative of no treatment at all. This information and these options must be conveyed to patients in a language and with terms they can genuinely understand. Patients denied access to such information and options cannot make reasonable choices, cannot be practically autonomous. Patients also have the right to make these reasonable choices as freely as possible. They have a right to accept or refuse medical care even when the choices they make are not those advised by their physicians. Obviously, their very sickness coerces them into choices they would otherwise not make. But the context of medical choice must be kept as otherwise free of coercion as possible, including the indirect coercions of offers of better care and facilities or better relationship with their physician. No one of us is absolutely free in our lives, but patients can achieve a meaningful level of practical freedom if those around them and caring for them respect their rights as persons. Beyond these rights, practical patient autonomy can generally be maximized if patients are helped and encouraged to learn more and choose better about their sicknesses and the paths open to increased wellness. As is usually the case in securing value beyond duty, such help and encouragement can not be specified here but must be left instead to the value creativity of the earnest professional in the concrete situation.

This demand for the right to informed consent, and for the values that take us beyond it, has had many recent critics who say that this concept is a legal innovation, or that it is practically irrelevant, or that most patients do not and will not assert such a right or express such an interest.[8] These criticisms are of little weight when one embraces the ideals we have chosen. If this is a new legal notion, then we may be heartened that the law has finally evolved to capture this much more of our moral demands. If patients cannot understand all the technical dimensions of their medical care, we can, nevertheless, take reasonable measures to insure that patients understand the general character of what is being done to them and why, and in layman's terms. If patients cannot be absolutely free, we can, nevertheless, take reasonable measures to insure practical freedom from coercion. Absolute personal autonomy is our ideal, but we must and can realize it in part in the world of fact. If most patients do not or will not exercise their rights, as with all rights, the having of them entails the right not to assert them as well. The day is likely coming, and it is not so distant, when patients will be far more knowledgeable about their medical care, far more willing and able to assert their free wills in medical contexts, and far more self-conscious of their autonomy and value as human persons. It behooves those involved with contemporary medical care to prepare for that day and to hasten its arrival, if they are to discharge the duties incumbent on them as professionals in a complex society. Our new knowledge and new power will be enslaving instead of liberating if we do not, and great potential for the maximization of practical personal autonomy will have been lost.

B. Patient Passivity, Cooperation, and Participation

With this perspective on the health care professional and his or her obligations towards patients in hand, let us look more closely at the character of the doctor-patient relationship and especially at its moral dimension.[9]

There appears to be basically three kinds of doctor-patient relationships; those in which the patient is passive to therapy, those in which the patient cooperates with therapy, and those in which the patient is an active participant in therapy. Of course, such distinctions are abstract and analytical. In most real relationships there will be elements of two or all of these models at different times and in different circumstances. Thus, factual doctor-patient relationships will often fall between these clear boundaries with all of the variety and nuance of any human relationship. Before characterizing each model further, it might be useful to think of these models as analogous to various stages in the parent-child relationship. Initially, the infant is wholly passive to the parents' care. Through childhood and adolescence cooperation between parent and child gradually increases. In ideal, child and parent arrive at a relationship of mutuality as adults. There are some important differences between these relationships and the models of the doctor-patient relationship as will become evident shortly, but a comparison with the analogous parent-child relationship is generally revealing.

In the most minimal relationship, the active-passive model, the doctor acts and the patient is acted upon. The physician relates to the patient as a parent to an infant. In the purest cases, the patient consciously contributes nothing to the success or failure of therapy. Even when the patient's body is treated with the utmost respect in this sort of a relationship, it takes on the character of an object, a thing for the ministrations of the physician. There are a variety of cases in which this is the most appropriate or the only possible relationship. Medical relationships with infants, with the unconscious, or with the mentally handicapped are of this minimal sort. It may also be the best model for most emergency medical care.

A fuller human relationship is achieved in the guidance-cooperation model. Here, the doctor commands and the patient obeys, the doctor leads and the patient follows. The doctor in this case is a frankly paternalistic guide and the patient, regardless of actual age, assumes the role of juvenile cooperator. While the patient here is no mere thing but a real party to the therapy, he or she is the decidedly dependent and unequal party. Perhaps such a patient follows a health regimen prescribed by the physician or takes medications at the intervals ordered, but the patient does not become a party to the decision-making itself. The doctor is deferred to completely in this. Here too there are situations in which this is the most appropriate therapeutic relationship or the fullest human one possible. Medical relationships with children, with senile adults, or with persons of low intelligence are examples. In the preparation for major medical procedures such as surgery and in the hospital care immediately afterwards, this may also be the most appropriate model.

The third and last model is that of mutual participation. In this model, doctor and patient are both conscious of their moral equality as persons, or at least potentially so. They relate to one another as two adults. The right of the patient to fully informed and free consent is recognized and respected by the physician. Trust, openness, and mutuality in decision-making are the hallmarks of this model. Both parties are aware of being involved in a joint venture, one potentially satisfying to both. In the cases of most adult, conscious, and relatively intelligent patients such a model is appropriate. It is also probably the most appropriate model for office visits and for the treatment of chronic and degenerative sicknesses.

It should be obvious that our ideal of the autonomous person requires that this last model of mutual participation be adopted whenever it is possible and to the extent that it is possible. It should stand as a regulative ideal for movement out of the other relationships, if such movement is factually possible. At times, this will be a natural movement, one very similar to the usual changes in the parent-child relationship. In an emergency room crisis, for example, an active-passive model may be the only one available. In the subsequent hospitalization, the relationship may advance to the guidance-cooperation model. Finally, as wellness becomes partially restored, the mutual participation model becomes appropriate. At times, there can simply be no advance. A highly dependent and immature adult, for example, may refuse to be treated as an adult and may cling instead to the security of the guidance-cooperation model, regardless of the best efforts of the physician. At times, the course of the models will reverse itself entirely as when the formerly mature adult slips into the guidance-cooperation model due to senility and then becomes wholly passive to the therapy of the doctor in the late stages of dying. Even in this case, if elements of the former more adult relationship can be salvaged in the guidance-cooperation model, they should be; and if elements of the guidance-cooperation model can be salvaged in the active-passive one, they should be too. For the same reasons that the mutual participation model is to be preferred over all, the guidance-cooperation model is to be preferred to the active-passive model. In both cases, protection of practical patient autonomy requires that the fullest human relationship of equality be achieved when the factual demands of the needed medical care themselves allow it, and so far as they allow it.

There are other good reasons for the moral priority of the mutual participation model. As the reason already given, protection of the autonomy of the patient, is an expression of our duty to treat all persons as equals, so these other reasons are expressive of the ethical challenges to enhance practical patient autonomy by maximizing full participation of the patient in the therapeutic relationship. These reasons are expressions of our commitment to values beyond duty.

The first additonal reason for preferring the mutual participation model arises out of some of the most profound changes that have occurred and will soon occur in contemporary medicine and in the biological sciences related to medicine. We are at the frontier of new medical interventions in the areas of behavior control, genetic engineering, control over sexual and even asexual reproduction, control over death through life support techniques that both extend life and the dying process. These and other exotic medical innovations of recent and approaching years add up to a biological and medical revolution. Against the social horizon of this revolution and the staggering range of human choices this revolution heralds, one can no longer speak about what is medically indicated without reference to social, political, and legal considerations, religious and ethnic backgrounds, and all of the ambiguities of individual moral choice. Achieving effective and humane medicine in such a context will require considerable openness and dialogue between doctor and patient, considerable sharing of information and decision-making, considerable deference to and support for patient autonomy. These are the strengths of the mutual participation model.

Secondly, the dramatic successes of medicine in the developed nations, and the equally dramatic success of efforts to improve sanitation, nutrition, and awareness of health risks, have led to a great decline in the incidences of sickness and death from infectious diseases in these nations. As a result of this success, chronic and degenerative diseases and those diseases most clearly related to life-style, including accidents, have come to make up a much larger percentage of these nations' morbidity and mortality rates. Effective and humane medicine designed to cope with these health problems will require the mutual participation model. Controlling chronic and degenerative diseases and advising on life-style questions will necessitate the sharing, openness, and autonomous participation of the patient.

Thirdly, there is evidence that suggests that mutual participation in the doctor-patient relationship makes for better, more effective medical care.[10] Patients in such medical relationships understand their conditions and how to improve them better than other patients, are more highly motivated to get better, and are more likely to follow their doctors' medical advice more faithfully. There are even recent claims that patients in such relationships tolerate pain better and recover from surgery faster.[11] If this evidence is reliable, then it is plain that these doctor-patient relationships are more medically effective than others. Clearly, it is in the interests of patients, physicians, and society as a whole that mutual participation models should prevail in medical contexts if they truly serve to make medicine a more effective tool for eliminating sickness and promoting wellness. The prevalence of this model would serve to minimize evil and maximize good.

A fourth consideration is the professional and human satisfaction of the physician. Our proper emphasis on the rights of patients should not obscure the fact that physicians and all members of the health care team are themselves incalculably great values as human persons. As such, the practical personal autonomy of each health care professional is a good which ought to be maximized. The physician who dictates a less than mutual participation relationship when such a relationship is possible, consigns himself or herself to relating to beings perceived as inferior or inconsequential persons. The attitude which displays itself in such remarks as "the kidney problem in Room 206" is its own punishment, as the bearer of such an attitude closes off the possibilities of cognitive and emotional growth for himself or herself by making fuller human interaction with patients less likely or impossible. By contrast, the forming of positive relationships between persons is, as we have seen, a key ingredient in building real autonomy. Only the model of mutual participation underscores the human worth of the patient and thus draws attention to this person as a source of value-creativity, a source from which there may be much for the physician to learn and to grow from.

Fifthly, we have already suggested that patients are very poor health care consumers and indicated some of the reasons why this is so. But patients, in spite of the barriers they face in making accurate judgments about the quality of their medical care, make these judgements in any case. Significant among the factors on which patients do make judgments is their perception of their physician's affective behavior, especially his or her perceived ability to feel and demonstate empathetic concern for patients. The chances for the existence and conveyance of such an emotional response seems greatest in a relationship of mutual participation wherein not only information and decisions are shared but, since they attach to all significant human discourse, emotions are shared as well. A physician may very well enhance his or her professional reputation in the eyes of patients and thus enhance the range of reasonable and free professional choices in his or her own career by developing a habit of forming this kind of therapeutic relationship.[12]

Finally, it is common knowledge that there is great consumer alienation from medical care at the social level.[13] Because of its greater reliance on impersonal machinery, because of the fragmentation of care inherent in medical specialization, because of the bureaucratic and business dimensions of hospital care, because of its cost, and because of the widespread perception that physicians just make too much money; for these reasons contemporary medicine is often accused of dehumanizing and even exploiting its patients. The existence of such attitudes on the part of the public is obviously not in medicine's interest; but it is not in the public's interest either, as cynicism about medical care will tend to make persons delay in seeking needed medical help. These delays can increase sickness and its associated pain, suffering, loss of autonomy, and negative self-consciousness. A wholesale institutional commitment by medicine to the mutual participation model might go a long way to help improve these public attitudes. By and large, medical professionals have unusually high ideals and the will and abilities to express those ideals in practice. Daily they save lives and reduce human suffering. Greater attention to the character of their relationships with patients in general would establish this fact more firmly in the public mind and would further secure the many goods which derive from contemporary medicine.

Not only, therefore, is the achievement of doctor-patient relationships marked by openness and the sharing of knowledge and decision-making a duty following from respect for the rights of patients, but it is also a way to maximize the achievement of significant human values for the benefit of patient, physician, and society alike. Thus, the widespread establishment of doctor-patient relationships of mutual participation would both satisfy the duty to avoid evil and at the same time would go beyond duty to maximize attainment of other important goods.

C. Doctors as Teachers and the Teaching of Doctors

The nature of the doctor-patient relationship as we have described it in ideal implies a role for doctors as teachers, a role suggested by the very name doctor itself (docere, to teach). Doctors, for example, give medical advice to their individual patients, and the giving of advice by an expert to a nonexpert is a form of teaching. Doctors routinely try to teach patients how to stay well and how to return to wellness when they are sick. Doctors teach the specifics of disease management when cure is not possible, detailing the steps necessary to limit the progress of disease and the gravity of sickness. They also teach patients how to use the health care system by making referrals to specialists, hospitals, and other persons and institutions.

Insuring that the patient has given a genuinely free and informed consent to treatment requires considerable teaching. The patient must be brought to understand the condition, the need for the proposed course of treatment, risks associated with it, and alternative courses of treatment, including none at all. Given the fact that many patients will have little or no prior knowledge of biology and medicine, they will have to be taught the necessary rudiments of these sciences by their physicians. A genuinely free and informed consent can only take place when a patient learns these rudiments in his or her own terms. This teaching need not be a line by line analysis of a legal consent form. Indeed, the consent form itself ought to be a mere legalistic confirmation of the exchange of information and consent which has already occurred throughout the relationship between doctor and patient. The signing of a consent form, where appropriate, should be the least significant act from the point of view of the practical personal autonomy which the right of informed consent is meant to guard and enhance. It can represent the self-conscious culmination of an act of teaching, but is seldom an act of teaching itself.

The medical profession as a whole also has an important teaching function to discharge in society. As has already been made clear, much of contemporary sickness is related, at least indirectly to life-style and to the personal habits that compose a life-style. A proper emphasis on prevention of disease and sickness requires that the medical profession make a serious and sustained effort to educate the public on the various health implications of personal and social habits, from diet and exercise programs, to smoking and drinking, to the demands of safety in working places and automobiles. This teaching assignment is a delicate one as we have suggested: Vigorous censure of sickness producing habits must be tempered by sympathy for the human persons victimized by these habits. Not every doctor need assume such a public teaching function; this is neither possible nor necessary. But if the organized medical profession does not speak out on these issues and encourage individual physicians to speak out in their localities, then, even if no specific duty to another person is transgressed, great goods that could have been attained by such public education will have been lost.

Physicians will also have to be teachers if we are to maximize the number of doctor-patient relationships of mutual participation. Considerable teaching must occur before the average person will be factually capable of assuming a relationship of mutual participation with a physician. There can be no denying, prior considerations notwithstanding, that many patients will in fact resist the challenges implied by such relationships. Many patients may continue to prefer to be told what to do by physicians in a frankly paternalistic manner. Old habits die slowly, and many contemporary patients have been habituated to defer to doctors. Also, the anxiety of sickness leads many patients to deify their doctors, to confer on them attributes of omniscience and omnipotence. With some of these patients, nothing can be done but to acquiesce to their immaturity. With others, however, effective and emotively reinforcing education by their physicians can lead them to a fuller participation with therapy. Where this teaching can be done, it ought to be done.

If doctors are to play this critical role as teachers even as they provide the best in scientific, machine supported medicine, they will themselves need to be educated with special care. There can be no turning back from the scientific and technological path of modern medicine; it is medicine's close association with science and technology that has made it the effective tool it is today. Doctors of tomorrow will need even more understanding of science and technology than those of this generation. In addition to these competencies, however, the attainment of relationships of mutual participation with patients and the teaching of both individuals and the public about health care will require that other goals become integrated into medical education as well.

First, medical students will have to be taught how to respect their patients' right to informed consent. Preliminary to this task is the need to convey to medical students the moral importance of this right as a protection of the autonomy of each patient. Next, language skills, skills tantamount to the ability to translate from one language to another, will need to be taught in medical schools if future doctors are to be able to explain complex scientific and technical details to their patients in terms patients can genuinely understand. This entails a honing of that intuitive grasp we all have more or less for "knowing" when we have been understood and when we have not. Finally, learning to respect a patient's right to informed consent means learning to refrain from dominating patients, a skill harder and harder to learn as the competition for entry into medical school builds a sense of elitism among those who are admitted, and as the power of modern medicine continues to grow.[14] Medical students must learn to accept the fact that the values they hold are not the only reasonable values in life and that because this is so, some of their patients will exercise the right to give or withhold consent to treatment in ways which they as doctors will find personally unacceptable. Neverthless, patient autonomy is only genuine and practical when patients are permitted to do what they conscientiously believe they must do, regardless of its medical advisability. These are hard but necessary lessons.

Secondly, future doctors must be taught how to feel concern for their patients and how to show that concern. Clearly, medical students also need to learn how to control their spontaneous emotional reactions to the pain, suffering, loss of autonomy, and death of their patients; at least insofar as these spontaneous emotions are near to raw passions. A doctor who weeps when alert and calculated action is called for serves no one's best interest. On the other hand, too good a control of the emotions on doctors' parts can lead to cold, impersonal medicine; a feeling already too much conveyed to patients by the mechanical and bureaucratic ambience of much contemporary medical care. A doctor who cannot weep for a patient has blunted an important dimension of his or her life as a human person and has closed off a significant avenue of communication and mutual sharing with patients. Medical students must be taught how and when to bring appropriate feelings into a medical relationship, feelings which will enhance care, improve healing, and stamp the doctor-patient exchange with the mark of the human.

Thirdly, along with the highest available standard of care, today's medical student must be taught the centrality of "first, do no harm." This means developing in medical students a spontaneous and deeply felt outrage at intuitively obvious cases of patient abuse and a commitment not to tolerate such abuses among their professional colleagues. What is seen to be wrong surely, directly, and without argument makes up the heart of a morality; cynicism, indifference, and overly fine argumentation can destroy morality. Of growing importance is the applicability of the "first do no harm" principle to life prolonging and death prolonging medical technologies. Just as medical students are taught when and how much of a drug to prescribe and when not to prescribe it, they must also be taught the more ambiguous but also most important skill of knowing how much therapy to prescribe for the dying, and especially when to prescribe no further aggressive therapy at all. Often it is the next of kin who will make such decisions, but since they just as often do so in light of the advise their physicians provide, medical students must know when to say enough is enough, when to advise that all active measures except care itself should cease. The variety of patients and their situations make a general rule on this issue hard to state, but surely aggressive therapy loses its human justification when death is proximate, inevitable, and accepted by the patient. Imposing or advising continued aggressive therapy in such a circumstance only prolongs the act of dying and thereby increases pain, suffering, and the compromise of patient autonomy.

This point itself entails that medical students must learn to accept the inevitability of their individual patient's pain, suffering, loss of autonomy, and deaths even as they actively fight against these evils. This, too, is a hard lesson and one which needs to be learned thoughout our society. The growing efficacy of medicine and media popularizations of them engender expectations among the public that something can always be done medically to effect a cure or at least a remission of disease. Because of the combative relationship between doctor and death, the loss of a patient can appear as a professional defeat for the individual doctor. Because of our cultural and personal denials of mortality, the acceptance of another's death can be an uncomfortable admission of the inevitability of one's own death for the physician and the next of kin alike. In spite of this, hospital dying will continue to appear and to be a human indignity if sound human judgments cannot be made about when to cease aggressive attempts to keep the obviously dying alive. These judgements are only possible when the inevitability of pain, suffering, loss of autonomy, and death is accepted.[15]

This need for sound human judgment brings us to a last goal for medical education. Before the middle of the twentieth century, medicine was filled with sound human judgment and little else. With the advent of scientific and technological medicine, machines are being increasingly relied upon to diagnose and to indicate appropriate treatment. But machines, as useful as they are, will never to able to replicate a contextual and intuitive moral judgment by a human being. Machines can only operate on rules and general principles and cannot feel and "know" when a rule or a principle needs suspension or alteration in the face of the needs of real persons in particular situations. Furthermore, questions of whether and how to use our new scientific and medical power cannot themselves be decided internal to science or medicine. Instead, both science and medicine must be regulated by human ideals and goals external to themselves, ideals and goals which assure that these new powers are used for the benefit of the persons and societies they were designed to serve. Medical students must be taught to understand and appreciate both the strengths and limitations of machine intelligence and when it needs to be overruled by a contextual moral choice. If medical students are not taught to impose human moral judgments on machine intelligence, future doctors and their patients will have machine intelligence imposed on them. It is unfortunate but true that the logic of technology in the twentieth century to this point has been inexorable: What can be done, is done.[16] Unless medicine can help to interrupt this logic with a judgment of what ought and ought not to be done, the use of technology in medicine will make us increasingly the slaves of our own machines.

Designing a medical education to include these goals will require that the human sciences, the humanities, and especially the study of ethics become integrated into the curricula of medical schools. This will inevitably mean a paring down somewhat of the present emphasis on science education. Obviously, no one benefits if medical education produces moral and compassionate physicians who are scientifically inept, so moves in this direction must be very circumspect and must make constant appeal to what dimensions of science are of most direct relevance to contemporary medical practice. Some curricular room might be created in medical schools if a greater effort were made thoughout our educational system to teach science as a method; a method of accurate observation, reasonable hypothesis formation, logical inference, and empirical test. Too often science is presented as a collection of facts. But these facts change, and in any case are readily available to practicing physicians in reference works and computers.[17]

Whether and how the human sciences, humanities, and ethics enter directly into the curricula of medical schools is secondary to the importance of an openness on the part of medical school faculty to their content. This is especially critical in the clinical training of third and four year medical students and residents. A whole course in medical ethics is probably not nearly as influential for medical students as the example of their clinical faculties' moral behavior. A great deal of medical practice is learned by observing and following the examples of faculty and practicing physicians. If the exemplars for tomorrow's physicians display respect for patient rights, affective concern, a commitment to avoiding harm, an acceptance of death, and a willingness to make hard moral judgments; if these attitudes establish the social horizon for the formation of a young doctor's habits, then many of the goals described here will be well served outside the formal curriculum.

In conclusion, it should be added that many of these same considerations are true of the educational needs of other health care professionals. Medicine is now clearly a team effort. It would be quite impossible as we know it without the contributions of nurses, dentists, pharmacists, medical technicians, and all the members of the various health professions. They too are educators in need of a special kind of education. This is especially so for nurses, since they are the most direct providers of patient care. It is the nurse who must mediate between the science and technology of contemporary health care and the human needs of individual patients. Though nurses, as all the other members of the health care team, are generally under the authority of physicians in their relationships with patients, nursing relationships are more sustained and regular then are the average physician's. In many cases, it is the nurse who further elaborates the patient's condition and choices, who provides the greatest emotional support, who sees that the patient is not harmed, who helps directly in the acceptance of sickness and death, and who aids in patient and next of kin decision-making. Because of this, most of what has been said about the needs of medical education are of equal weight for nursing education.[18] And here there is one further point. There is probably no one better situated in contemporary medicine to take on the role of advocate for patients' rights than the nurse. Such advocacy may involve direct expressions like asserting a patient's interests to doctors and hospital personnel or indirect expressions like informing patient and family that the patient does indeed have rights which must and will be respected if claimed. In either case, and in a myriad of cases in between, the contemporary nurse is in a unique position to have a significant influence in determining whether the medicine of tomorrow will be as humane as it is technically effective. Nurses must be educated to accept and perform this critically important humanizing role.

Chapter 9.

The Child Patient

A. Children's Rights

Our discussion of the sick person, the health care professional, and the nature of the relationships that should arise between them has largely focused on the conscious, intelligent adult, someone capable of having and interested in securing a therapeutic relationship of mutual participation. Once again we have begun with the ideal case and must now recognize some of the more difficult cases that arise in fact. What are the implications for this position if the patient is unconscious, low in intelligence, or someone incapable or uninterested in having an adult therapeutic relationship? Some of the most important of these implications can be made plain if we focus on the cases in which the patient, by definition, is not an adult. Let us examine the general features of the new moral issues which arise when the patient is a child.

The point has already been made that although it is the value creative activity of the self that is the source of our notion of practical personal autonomy and human rights, it is our species as a whole which bears the possibilities for such individual achievements in our collective genetic and cultural inheritances. Thus species membership, as defined by the best available science, is the widest, most progressive criterion for the indentification of potentially autonomous persons and thus bearers of human rights. Such a broad criterion and goal will allow for a sensitivity to all human rights claims without arbitrary exception. Though it has not been part of this task to explore them, there are likely additional moral demands on persons and societies which restrict our freedom of action with respect to animals, plants, and the environment as a whole. Certainly it is a mark of prudence at the very least to encourage habits of respect toward all forms of life, and the general conditions for life as we know it. There is pleasure and pain in the animal world generally, and intimations of happiness and suffering among the more developed mammals. We cannot be morally callous to the pains and sufferings we often inflict on animals. But there appears to be nothing in the plant or animal worlds or in the environment in general which mirrors the value creative activity of the human species. Thus our most compelling moral demands center on the values and duties found in our relationships with individual human persons in our species.

It is important to insist that, having embraced this progressive criterion for identifying persons, the rights of all members of our species must be considered equal. This is so because of our ideal of the human person and the possibilities for practical personal autonomy inherent in that ideal. It is not so due to any degree of factual realization of practical personal autonomy in any given case. Thus the determination of the rights of persons in the ideal makes direct reference to ideals only and not to fact. This is part of the morally radical nature of our general thesis. Differences among persons in factual skills, strengths, moral virtue, even in practical personal autonomy are irrelevant to the having of equal human rights; instead one has equal human rights solely on the basis of species membership. Consider the alternatives here. Were we to say that some but not all members of our species are persons with rights, we should have to produce some nonarbitrary justification for why some human beings are to be considered persons and some are not. Producing such a nonarbitrary justification has proven to be as difficult in theory as it is dangerous in fact. Or, if we were to admit that all human beings have some rights but that these rights vary on the basis of some factual individual achievements such as intelligence, virtue, age, etc., we shall have an equally difficult time justifying our selection of rights making characteristics and of identifying their fullness in practice. Who will be smart enough to have rights, for example, and how will we clearly determine it? Whose virtue is sufficient to guarantee his or her human rights, and can we objectively measure it? And if we do use the existence of any factual ability or virtue to determine a person's rights, we will have the additional problem of having to account for our intuitive respect for a person's rights even when that person is not expressing that ability or virtue as in cases of sleep, intoxication, coma, senility, irrationality, viciousness, etc. This moral intuition suggests that it is not the factually real having of any ability or virtue which makes for rights but one's ideal status itself. If, instead of any factual ability or virtue, age is taken to be the criterion for the having of equal rights; what is the right age to have the rights of a human person, and why not one year, one month, or one minute earlier? As practically needful as age limits are for the having of some legal rights, from the moral point of view, age limitations on human rights appear arbitrary. In spite of the difficulties inherent in our identification of all members of the human species as persons having equal rights, these difficulties seem minor compared with the difficulties implied both theoretically and practically by these alternatives.

If all members of the human species are persons with equal rights, then children have equal rights, too. They are persons and, regardless of age, have the same human rights as any and every other person. Children do not have fewer rights or partial rights. They are not developing or growing into their rights. They do not have to wait to learn to reason, to develop a sense of themselves, to be practically autonomous, or to achieve any factual expression of value creative activity whatsoever in order to have human rights. Children have rights by virtue of the same criterion you or I do, by virtue of membership in the human species.[1] I do not inspect the factual details of your value creative activities as a person to determine whether or not you have rights, nor do you inspect mine. I may be indifferent to some of your deepest held values, or they may even be repugnant to me, and vice versa. The factual specifics are irrelevant; identification of another being as a member of our species is the only factual determination

110

that needs to be made before rights arise which ought to be respected. Similarly, it is not inspection of the immature factual value creative activity of children that establishes their rights. In the extreme cases of infants and the comatose in terminal illness, there is little or no value creative activity, yet there are still rights. Our respect for factual value creative activity in these cases is only by expectation or by memory, but our respect for the rights of those involved is by virtue of their being human persons, members of our species. In like manner, children have complete and equal human rights regardless of the degree of their factual attainments.

But clearly these are assertions of the ideal. As a matter of fact, children, especially very young children, cannot claim their rights.[2] Without the factual ability to assert claims about rights and to have those assertions respected by others, the factual ability to enjoy rights will be extremely curtailed among children. Children, therefore, are factually dependent on adults to assert their rights for them. Thus there is a profound bond of trust between adults and children. Children are equal to adults in value and rights in the ideal but need the factual commitment of adults to even approach that ideal in reality.

This tension between having rights in the ideal and not being able to assert them for oneself in fact has a contradictory air about it. That a child both is and is not a complete person is a mark of the rapid developmental period that childhood most essentially is. But this is a tension expressive of a wider phenomenon: It is characteristic of all growth, of all process. An acorn as it grows both is and is not an oak tree at any given time. A melody as it is played both is and is not before the mind at once. A person entering into and concluding relationships with others both is and is not free at any moment. Everything that develops both is and is not. In this light, a child is a person in process; person full and complete in ideal, yet partial and incomplete in fact.

This process of childhood, of growing into factual personhood, is known to be highly vulnerable both physically and culturally. The future real person of the present child can be severely impaired physically by lack of adequate nutrition, clothing, housing, health care, etc. The future real person of the child can also be dwarfed culturally by lack of affection, parental guidance, literacy, education in general, etc. Thus we know that there is a relatively clear set of minimal conditions which must obtain for a child to grow from factual dependencies into a practically autonomous adult. Children have a right to these conditions. Children have equal human rights in the ideal but, due to their empirical vulnerability in common and highly structured relationships with adults, special rights arise for children. Thus far from having fewer rights, children, in a sense, have more; not numerically more rights, but the same human rights articulated against a background of conditions known to jeopardize the realization of a practical measure of autonomy in fact. Children have rights to be free from those conditions known to impair development toward adulthood, and rights of access to those things and conditions known to be necessary

111

to develop toward adulthood. As adults have rights to have their autonomies protected, so children have rights to have their processes of autonomy development protected as well.[3]

This situation raises special challenges for pediatric medicine. The child patient, as a bearer of full and equal human rights, deserves the same therapeutic relationship of mutual participation, so far as he or she is able. On the other hand, the child by definition will seldom be able to enter into such a relationship. Our regulative goal stands, however: So far as the child is factually able to understand and rationally choose, he or she should be permitted to do so. Of course, determining whether and to what extent any particular child is able to choose will be a contextual judgment on the part of pediatrician and parent. Surely no elements of this relationship are available to infants and to very young children. On the other hand, a large part, perhaps all of the mutual participation model, is possible with a mature teenager. It is in the developing years between infancy and teenage that the difficulty is most acute practically, but the principle remains clear even here. Children should be made participants in their care so far as they are able and so far as it is not medically dangerous. This last qualification must be added to cover cases in which a child might be intellectually mature enough to be able to grasp the nature of the sickness but whose emotional immaturity is such that frank information might jeopardize his or her long term best interest. There is a wide and morally necessary range of choices which parents and other adults must make for a child's own best interest when the child cannot choose for himself or herself. This paternalism is justified by the peculiar combination of the child's ideal nature and factual immaturity. However, if a child is to grow into a full measure of practical autonomy as an adult, the immature child must be brought into decisions as early and as often as possible. This is education for autonomy and there is no substitute for it.

When the child cannot be meaningfully involved in his or her own care, and especially when the child cannot practically exercise the right to informed consent, the child's right to participate and give or withhold informed consent passes to a third party who exercises it for the child.[4] This third person has a proxy or substituted right to choose for the child, but also the consequent duty to do so only in the best interests of the child. Normally, this third party will be the child's parent or parents, guardian, or next of kin. Because of the natural and deeply felt emotive bond between child and parent or parent substitute, this practical transfer of the child's rights makes obvious good sense and is generally exercised on behalf of what is clearly in the best interest of the child. When this is not the case, however, other adults must intervene to see to it that the child's rights are respected in the medical context. If it seems to make little sense to assume that such a strong emotive bond exists, as in the case of a parent who has long since effectively abandoned his or her child, or it becomes evident that the parent is choosing not for the child but for the parent's own selfish interests; in such cases, the parent has lost the moral right to choose for the child. Parents have no absolute right to choose for their children because children are not things which can be owned. Though children belong to their parents, parents do not own their children. Only things can be owned. Only with things, and only sometimes even here, can we operate with wholly selfish motives, with indifference to the perspective of the thing. Children belong to their parents only so that parents can help to insure that they grow into and realize as much of their ideal autonomy as they are factually capable of realizing. When parents clearly thwart this process, their children no longer belong to them morally and other adults must intervene on behalf of these children.

This duty to intervene for the child and against a parent or parent substitute is a general duty owed by all adults to all children and is based on the demand that we respect equal human rights. This duty places special hardship on a pediatrician when he or she discovers child abuse or neglect, or when a parent refuses needed medical procedures or opts for unnecessary medical procedures for a child; that is, when the pediatrician earnestly believes that a parent is choosing to serve his or her own interests and not the child's. In such cases, the pediatrician must intervene on behalf of the child and must use the force of the legally protected rights of the child if necessary. Coming between a parent and a child in this manner will never be easy but there are cases in which it must be done to protect the primary right of the child.[5] And here as elsewhere, when our morality and our ethical reflections demand it, we must create humane and effective institutions and practices to facilitate at the social level the protection of childrens' rights both in and out of medical contexts.

B. Dependence and the Sick Child

Part of the challenge implied by this theory of the ideal and fact worlds is that of showing how the ideal world can make demands on us without qualification and, at the same time, how those moral demands must meet and engage the world of fact. This challenge is graphic when considering the case of children whose ideal nature makes them equal and incalculably valuable persons but whose factual situation makes them extremely vulnerable before and dependent upon others. In order to see more fully the moral realities of values and duties in our relationships with children, we must further explore their factual dependencies.

Children are directly dependent on their biological parents for their genetic inheritance. For the individual child, the union of his or her parents' germ cells fixes once and for all a multitude of facts and possibilities for the child's life. A given child may inherit a body and personality prone to wellness; another is sickly from the start. Notice the obvious here. These facts about children happen to them beyond their control and beyond any intelligible use of the category of merit. No child deserves his or her parents or the body that has resulted from their sexual union. This is the truth in the juvenile complaint, "I didn't ask to be born." No one of us did; nor did we ask for the specific circumstances into which we were born. Here we must speak again of luck, good and bad.

The chance character of our bodies and our births forever affects our lives, as the body we begin with determines the outlines of our physical futures, and as the time, place, and circumstances of our births determine the outlines of our social futures. We all begin most intimately tied to facts we did not, and perhaps would not, choose for ourselves.

Children are directly dependent on their mothers for proper biological development during gestation. It is now clear scientifically that the adequate diet of a mother during pregnancy is crucial in determining her child's chances of being born with a strong body and a well developed brain.[6] Where there are high rates of maternal illness and consequently high rates of fetal malnutrition as in the developing nations, there are also high rates of infant mortality. These rates can take on tragic proportions. In some developing nations, infant mortality runs as high as 8 to 10 times that of some of the more developed nations; preschool mortality runs up to 30 times as high.[7] Further, the inability of the mother or father to secure proper nutrition for the child in infancy can lead to permanent impairments directly and to others indirectly through an increase in the malnourished child's susceptibility to infectious and parasite borne diseases. Thus we see once again that the child's future is shaped in dramatic ways by events over which the child has no control; whether or not the child's mother was herself nourished and adequately cared for during gestation, and whether the mother or anyone else could secure a proper diet for the child in the fragile months and years immediately after birth.

The child after birth is shaped by a host of parental choices, many of which are so spontaneously emotive and habitual as to be unconscious.[8] Perhaps the most permanent stamp on a child comes from the emotive climate of the household. Many factors, including whether a child was initially wanted or not, can shape the affective environment as the child grows. The parents' choices of clothing, housing, and education have a direct effect on the child's wellness, physical and mental. The habits of the household make an impress second only to that of nature itself. Until a more mature perspective develops, the child's world is experienced through the family the way the adult world is experienced through body and mind, i.e. transparently. The family is the world of experience, and what is right and proper in the family just is right and proper absolutely. The emotions and habits of the family make the household a powerful vehicle for shaping the child's worldview, again the child has little or no control. And it must be added that many of the parents' choices are beyond their own conscious control as well. Fixed habits blind parents to alternatives, and social circumstances like poverty, unemployment, scarcity of food, and poor parental education, may dictate their choices for them.

Finally, the child is dependent on the culture into which he or she is born. Our cultures set our life's horizons for us, determining in large part our interpretations of the past, expectations for the future, and sense of place in the present. While the child may grow into a critical adult perspective on culture, the child as child knows no world but that which parents and culture present — with culture shaping the parents' perspective as well. To appreciate the importance of this point, consider the factual impact on a child born into a culture of small cohesive social units such as a small town, a tribe, or an ethnic community surrounded by other groups. Compare this to the factual impact of birth and development in a large metropolitan area of multiple but shallow relationships and periodic relocations. For even more graphic examples, think of how one's life might be factually shaped if one has the misfortune of being born a member of the oppressed race in a racist society or the excluded gender in a sexist society. These factors and a multitude more too numerous and obvious to name establish the facts of our early lives. These early facts continue to shape us throughout our entire lives. Again, the inability of the child, any child, to direct these factors makes the child's progress toward practical personal autonomy dependent on forces beyond his or her rational control.

If we are to take our ideals of human equality and human rights seriously we must engage these factors. If a child cannot meaningfully realize autonomy unless potential parents understand the various health demands of pregnancy, then protecting the rights of the child means educating potential parents properly in this respect. If a child cannot factually approach the ideal of personal autonomy unless his or her mother had access to a proper diet for the child's early formative years, then respect for the rights of the child demands that society make that diet available and its critically important nature known to all mothers. If the parents' choices and the entire world of culture factually shape a child and determine the real possibilities of personal autonomy, then parents must be educated to the autonomy debilitating character of some of these choices and be provided with the means to avoid them.

There are many complex factual issues implied here. Competing social values and traditions will always and strongly come into play when one suggests criticism and change of habitual and deeply felt child rearing practices and of social habit in general. Nevertheless, it is a part of our ideal of a progressive society that it shapes its social habits in such a way as to allow for change in the direction of ever fuller realization of its ideals. It is tragic but true that for many persons, any possibility for the enjoyment of real practical personal autonomy was destroyed by early childhood. Respect for the rights of all persons, but especially for children, demands that we address the factors that destroy these possibilities and that we vigorously try to amend them to allow all human beings the fullest possible factual enjoyment of their ideal rights as persons. Simply put, it is our duty to protect the development of a child's autonomy. And here as elsewhere the ideals and ethical theory we have chosen will take us beyond this duty to steps that will actively enhance this developmental process for the individual child and for all children.

115

To draw these insights closer to medicine, we should now consider the additional factual dependencies of the sick child. Sickness as we understand it here is the self-conscious and negative fixation on an emergent body and mind or both, a fixation usually consequent on pain, suffering, or loss of practical personal autonomy. Sickness of any sort in a child is an emotionally poignant event for the child and for the adults who witnesses it. Not only does a serious childhood sickness threaten lifelong impairment and the possibility of death before human life has even matured, but childhood sickness appears to be an experience worse in itself then similar sickness in adults. The very nature of childhood makes this so.[9]

Compared to the average adult perception, the child is largely ignorant of the operations of the body and especially of the causes and remedies for pain. Ignorance may sometimes be bliss, but most sick adults take comfort from the knowledge of the causes of their pains and the expectation that something is generally available to palliate them. Adults can then place their pains into a larger cognitive framework; knowing, for example, that some injury that hurts keenly now will not hurt at all momentarily and is just not that medically serious. A young child knows only the pain without the assurance, without the cognitive framework. At the same time, the will of a child is weak by the nature of the case; if will is strengthened through habit, the ill formed habits of a child makes for a weak will. Thus the child cannot as easily embrace a painful but necessary exercise or accept a distasteful but needed drug on the sheer weight of will as most adults can. Because of these underdeveloped capacities of knowledge and will, the sick child is less capable of reasserting any measure of practical autonomy. The sick adult can take some measure of practical control over elements of a sickness. Seldom can the child do so.

It is also obvious that the emotions of a child, having been less educated by contact with reason, are closer to raw passions than are the emotions of the typical adult. Since raw passion is a spontaneous animal response to stimuli, the sick child is more prone to weep, scream, be overcome and carried away with strong and confused passions. The very ravages of these passions can bring suffering as the child, for example, is unable to keep from crying or screaming. And, of course, the very same lack of knowledge discussed above, combined with the energy of nearly raw passions, can drive the sick child to fears, misconceptions, and anxieties with a force not generally experienced by adults.

Behind these evident facts of childhood lie two others which shape childhood sickness in specific and substantial ways. In the first case, the child has a very underdeveloped and dramatic sense of self.[10] Ironically, the underdevelopment of the child's sense of self may be in part a function of the apparent fact that very young children move through experience as if everything were the self or its extension. Only gradually, through the resistances of their natural and social environments, do children begin to pare down this enlarged self to a conception more recognizably adult. The adult distinguishes more clearly between the self and the nonself and thus can more easily attribute causation and responsibility to factors outside the self; thereby freeing the self from blame where appropriate. The child cannot do so. At the same time the consciousness of a small child is typically dramatic and animistic. The child sees events as played out especially for him or her and usually with rewards and punishments from godlike forces like parents, older siblings, adults, and perhaps even by God in the case of an older child with a religious consciousness. Living with the self in so many things, and living with it so dramatically, can lead the sick child to a fixated negative self-consciousness more pervasive and punitive than that typically experienced by the adult. The sick child may see the world as sick and feel that this state of affairs is all his or her fault. The intensity of the feeling bad of the sick child may therefore be both wider and deeper than that of the sick adult. Such a consciousness can be felt and suffered from well before anything like it can be articulated. Because it cannot be described by the small child, the existence of this worsened sickness state is speculative. But if this account is broadly accurate, it would help to explain some of the sick child's emotive overreactions and some of the adult caretaker's feelings of special empathy.

We also know that children have great difficulty in coming to grips with time concepts and the words for them. The meaning of yesterday, tomorrow, last year, next month, etc., entirely escapes the young child. No doubt this apparent lack of a developed time consciousness is related to the child's confused sense of self; since our adult sense of self is a function of memories of the self in the past, anticipations of the self in the future, and the felt continuity of these selves with the one who is me in the present. With a very short personal past for memories and an impoverished ability to foresee the likely character of the future, children live in a world that is now. Promises of prevention of future sickness, wellness, or release from pain are largely empty and meaningless to the sick child. Equally, reference to past medical success can reasure little when one's memory is short. The sick child therefore does not have the mental refuges of the past and the future; delighting in memories of healthier days or anticipating renewed wellness are closed to a being who knows only the sickness felt today.

All of these facts or apparent facts must animate and modulate the application of our ideals to reality. If children in general have special vulnerabilities, then special rights arise for protection of those vulnerabilities: rights of freedom from destruction of the potential for autonomy and rights of access to those goods and services known to be necessary for approaching a realization of this ideal. If sick children have special needs because of the intensity of their sicknesses, then a commitment to maximizing the attainment of human values will compel us to address those specific needs in the medical context.[11] Steps must be taken to help the sick child know more and choose better, moderate feelings, and mitigate the negative consequences of undeveloped senses of self and of time. The facts of a child's sickness creates special needs; in these circumstances the moral ideal of personal autonomy creates for adults special duties to discharge and special values to attain. The central special duty is to work towards the day when sickness will not prevent any child from having a meaningful chance to realize a full measure of pleasure, happiness, and practical personal autonomy. The central value when dealing with childhood sickness is the moral mandate to create those actions and habits of action which will enhance childhood wellness and maximize the number of children who can live through their bodies and minds without self-conscious and negative fixation on them. The duty is to avoid the harms of childhood sickness. The value is to maximize the number of practically autonomous adults by insuring widespread childhood wellness.

C. Adults as Children

Attention to the special circumstances of the sick child illustrates the application of our moral ideals to some of the variety of the concrete world of fact. Similar results apply to cases of adults with diminished capacities for the realization of practical personal autonomy. The general principle in all such cases is the same: Factual barriers to the realization of practical personal autonomy must be removed and factual necessities for the realization of practical personal autonomy must be provided. These conclusions follow from the demands of recognizing our moral ideals' relevance to the world of fact as interpreted through our autonomy maximization ethics.

Perhaps the closest adult analogue to the situation of the sick child is the mentally handicapped adult. Obviously, our first duty here is to prevent these handicaps from occurring so far as we are able. Once again this will entail public educational efforts related to the causes and prevention of mental handicaps. It may also entail provision of adequate diet and health care to all pregnant women and certainly to those thought to be in danger of bearing a mentally handicapped child because of genetic reasons or because of the previous birth of such a child. The demands of care for these children after birth and throughout their lives as adults will vary as widely as the nature of the handicaps involved and the circumstances that these persons find themselves in.[12] The principle governing all of these efforts should be the achievement of as much functional autonomy as possible or, where little or no autonomy is possible, as much happiness and pleasure the mentally handicapped person is capable of enjoying.

Physically handicapped adults have different needs. Part of the great suffering caused by a severe physical handicap, especially a permanent one, is that the adult who thus suffers still has a full measure of personal autonomy in his or her ability to consciously reflect and to make free life choices. The inability to readily fulfill these reasoned choices in physical action must then be a consuming frustration. The knowledge that satisfaction of one's intentions depends not on the immediacy of body response as in the normal case, but on the continued good will and attention of others; this knowledge has the power in itself to generate an intensely fixated and negative self-consciousness. Acknowledging the equal rights of the physically handicapped means providing whatever services are necessary to allow them the fullest use of their physical environment possible given their individual conditions. Only in this manner can an intact mental autonomy direct itself meaningfully to its natural object, that is, to action in the physical world.

There are a multiplicity of human and health care needs that arise in old age. The elderly experience a decline in mental and physical powers, a decline which often reduces them to conditions not unlike that of children with one important exception. The incapacities of the child are real but they have a lighthearted, even comic dimension because of our confidence that time and maturity will bring the child to a fuller expression of human capacities. Thus the future is a field of hope for the child. In the case of the declining elderly, the comedy of capacities not yet developed is exchanged for the poignancy of capacities lost. Hope, at least as far as it is focused on the natural world, diminishes as the elderly witness their own skills fade and their relatives and friends pass away. In such a factual situation, the maximization of practical personal autonomy demands that every effort be made to preserve as much autonomy for the elderly for as long as possible. Here too the connections between personal autonomy as free and rational choice and the background of emotions and habits from which these choices emerge must not be overlooked. The availability of multiple and affectively supportive human contacts and of opportunities for continuing to build satisfying habits of work and play are crucial in sustaining the practical personal autonomy of the aged.

In the final period of decline, the elderly become the dying. The dying have special rights because of their extreme circumstances. Even before the notion of rights existed expicitly, there was still widespread recognition of the moral demands which the dying place on the living. Those in the dying process command our immediate attention and concern. Typically, we acquiesce to their every reasonable wish. Even when measures to prolong life have clearly failed, the dying have a right to continued efforts by the living to care for and comfort them right up to the end. The most important right of the dying in contemporary medical contexts is the right to be able to accept death on their own terms.[13] This entails a right to refuse aggressive medical therapies which merely extend the process of meeting an inevitable, proximate, and accepted death. Aggressive medical therapies lose their moral justification when they cease to prolong life and begin instead to prolong death. There is a growing fear, among the elderly in particular but throughout American society, that contemporary medicine will refuse to allow one to die one's own death in terms of one's own values. Many worry that, in spite of their wishes, aggressive medical therapies will be applied to prevent death; yet these therapies will not renew life, but merely incarcerate the dying person in a twilight or outright vegetative state. The having of a right of informed consent to medical treatment entails that the terminally ill have the right to designate in advance of death which therapies and resultant states of nonlife they find unacceptable and therefore refuse. Health care professionals and next of kin should feel morally bound by these demands whether written or oral. The ideal or personal autonomy becomes dreadfully attenuated in fact if it is robbed from us in the midst of one of life's most intimate of moments, at death itself.

This is emphatically not an assertion of a right to suicide nor is it "playing God." It cannot be suicide to accept a death one did not bring on oneself, especially when one has already accepted all reasonable measures to restore a meaningful human life. While hope of some medical cure may always be an abstract possibility, in the lives of real persons facing real events, there are times when hope in the natural world has no basis in fact. Unless we acknowledge the right to refuse death prolonging therapies, we will be forced into the absurdity of only being allowed to die from what medicine cannot cure, regardless of whether that medically permitted death is more painful, horrible, or compromising of the autonomy of the person than other more natural deaths. In such an absurd state of affairs medical technology imposes its own logic on us entirely and the human goals which regulated the very creation of this technology are lost sight of completely.

Furthermore, how can accepting an inevitable and proximate death be "playing God" when such acceptance has marked the conscious dying of most persons through human history, except for some persons in the developed nations for the last fifty years or so? Indeed, this charge may fairly be reversed and laid at the door of those who would continue aggressive therapy until there are no machines left to use. Surely it is more appropriate to say that one arrogates the power of God by frustrating indefinitely a natural occurrence, an occurrence which from a religious perspective may well be considered God's will itself.[14] By contrast, it is the wholly secular consciousness which sees no possibility of life beyond the natural that is most frenzied in the fact of death, most driven to deny the inevitable, most prepared to exchange the quality of a real human life for the quantity of machine supported nonlife. The maintenance of "life" in a human corpse is an indignity which assaults personal autonomy at the core, a personal autonomy which many religious traditions find central to their own beliefs. The preservation of practical personal autonomy up to the very end of human life whether for moral or religious reasons means respecting the demands of the terminally ill to die with dignity; and more than anything else this demand for a death with dignity is the demand to be allowed to die under conditions consistent with one's own values. To be forced to die under conditions dictated by someone else's values, especially if those values are exclusively those of a scientific and bureaucratic rationality, is the ultimate loss of autonomy. Alternately, assuring oneself a death accepted with dignity is the final natural act of the self's value creative activity. Every persons has a right to this.

These and related consideration could be and need to be articulated throughout the whole range of actual circumstances which affect the possibilities for persons achieving real autonomy. These observations show, it is hoped, that the ideals of personal autonomy and of equal human rights are not abstract and empty but are concrete challenges which must be brought into reality with a clear sense of fact and a broad sympathy for the human condition in all its variety. Again in these cases, we must discover our duties and create the conditions for the attainment of new values, values related to our human drives for pleasure, happiness, and practical personal autonomy.

There is a paradox in our attitudes toward children and adults that must be noted before we leave this topic. Our analysis has had the general structure that adults have certain rights and needs, but that children, because of their vulnerable growing processes, have more rights and greater needs; that certain categories of adults are like children in this respect; and that the factual diminution of the capacities for autonomy of these adults requires that we take special steps to insure that they too have a reasonable chance of attaining practical personal autonomy. But if we are to truly engage that fact world, we must admit that, arguments in the ideal for personal autonomy notwithstanding, many adults are factually like children in most respects and all adults are factually like children in some respects.

All of us as adults live through the bodies that grew with us as children and the physical limitations discovered or created then are carried far into adulthood, sometimes permanently. This same point is even stronger when said of the emotions. The good feelings and the bad, the deep satisfactions and the emotional scars, the education which our passions received or did not receive in childhood; all of these carry over and color adult emotional life. The habits of youth, if not the same as those of the adult, were the ones which set the conditions for the possibility of forming the habits that are the adult's. The reasonings and the choices of childhood open and close adult possibilities and shape forever the cognitive and attitudinal stance one takes toward the world. The child, to paraphrase an old saw, is the parent of the adult. Throughout the greater part of this self-parenting, the child was not at all or not fully a practically autonomous person. For most of us, the practical autonomy of our adult life shades ever so gradually out of the factual dependencies of childhood and for some of us, because of factors largely beyond our rational control, that shading of degrees never quite reaches a practically autonomous adulthood.

There are many moral implications here, but the most obvious implication for our purposes is that when factual circumstances tend to compromise the real attainment of autonomy even among well adults, those circumstances need to be addressed as well. When lack of personal freedoms make meaningful autonomy impossible, even for well adults, we must criticize and change the institutions and practices which stifle personal freedom. When scarcity of life's necessities such as food, housing, meaningful employment, health care, and education make practical personal autonomy impossible even for well adults, we are morally bound to criticize and change the social habits which bring these evils about. Adults, like children, are shaped by events, many of which are out of an individual person's control. Adults, like children, are in a process of continued growth through those events, one less dramatic and therefore less visible, but a process nevertheless. This process can be facilitated or frustrated in its orientation toward pleasure, happiness, and practical personal autonomy by factors which can only be addressed at the social level, and only freely and rationally so in a progressive society. Some of these necessary measures we will be duty bound to discover, others we will be driven to create beyond duty. In either case, we must recognize the factual dependencies of even the most autonomous of adults on the political and social habits within which he or she chooses and acts.

One final moral implication of the sameness and difference of children and adults is pertinent. There are many ways to clarify moral intuitions. Our way has been primarily cognitive. A very interesting emotive clarification is also easily available and quite useful in morally significant dealings with other adult persons such as those which routinely occur in health care contexts. When confused as to the depth and extent of your duties and values with respect to some adult person, try to envision this adult as a child. Acknowledge and respect his or her right to make autonomous decisions, of course, indeed encourage this. But at the same time imagine that these would-be rational choosings are issuing from the boy or girl this adult once was, the boy or girl who is habitually dependent, emotively fragile, and not at all sure of his or her place in the world. Not only does this technique enrich the ability to empathize with others, but it also provides a fundamental insight about all persons. Our practical personal autonomies are imperfect realities constructed not only on our moral ideals but also on the factual successes and failures of our individual childhoods, successes and failures that were and are largely out of our rational controls.

IV. Using the Tools: Some Social Dimensions of Medical Care

Chapter 10.

Hospitals

A. Institutionalizing Care and Cure

The ideal of personal autonomy has been the keystone of our approach to morality and ethics and to personal relationships in the medical context. Practical personal autonomy in decision-making is the ability to make rational choices and thus transcend one's circumstances and limitations in an act of freedom. As central expressions of the value creativity of the self, autonomy and the consequent ability to freely transcend oneself, are at the heart of our valuation of the self as incalculably great and are thus the core elements of human dignity. On this account it is because of our spontaneous, though historically incomplete, deference to this autonomous self-transcendence of the incalculably worthy self that we have developed an intuitively felt duty to respect the rights of persons and an equally intuitively felt drive to maximize the attainment of those values most directly significant for all persons. Our ethical formulation of this felt morality requires us to acknowledge and respect the equal rights of all human beings to freedom from interference with their liberties and to freedom of access to the goods and services necessary for a minimally acceptable human life. Within the constraints of this goal, our ethical principle requires us to seek to maximize the attainment of the human values of pleasure, happiness, and practical personal autonomy.

Attention to the fact world has led us to adjust and specify these ideals so that they can become tools for the improvement of reality. One of the most significant facts we have asserted is that the human person is inherently social. Though the private self alone experiences its own inwardness and subjectivity, the possibility and character of this experience is a function of our social nature. From our inheritance of the genetic structure of the brain to our inherited emotional education and factual abilities to reason, the human person is a social accomplishment. Human beings as members of a biological species are natural objects, but human persons as members of society are cultural achievements. Human beings in a species become human persons in a society when the fact world of the former becomes infused and enlivened by the ideal world of the latter. Only then can the value creativity of the self individuate a person through the unique ideals and values which that self embraces. As individuals we are each unique and irreplaceable, but that uniqueness and irreplaceability is built on the accumulated experience of the societies within which we each grow and develop. There can be little doubt that a certain kind of person is produced by a certain kind of society: martial societies produce military leaders; religious societies produce priests and prophets; commerical societies produce traders; mobile societies produce transient citizens. The mechanism for this fitting of person and society is clearly exhibited in child rearing practices, as parents seek to reinforce or extinguish behaviors and attitudes in the child with reference to standards absorbed from the parents' own social experience. Autonomous choice enters into the parenting process as well and this gives rise to individuality in children. But even the fullest practical personal autonomy only allows one to choose from the range of choices which are given and are perceived as reasonable; and one's society is centrally involved in shaping the given options for choice and one's perceptions of what is reasonable.

Sensitivity to this social dimension and especially to the ways in which it can significantly affect a person's real attainment of practical autonomy has led us to a companion ideal to that of personal autonomy, viz., the ideal of a progressive society. Such a society has its institutions and practices, i.e. its social habits, structured in such a way that continual social transcendence is allowed for, even encouraged. This will be an expression of what we might call social autonomy, the ability of a society to make free and reasonable collective choices through its institutions and practices. As we have seen, a fundamental condition for the development of a progressive society is democracy.

Democratic social habits help to assure the attainment of social autonomy because they allow for, and encourage, the widest possible citizen participation under the freest of conditions. The widest possible citizen participation, though it cannot guarantee the reasonableness of a public conclusion, at least guarantees that no point of view is excluded from consideration on principle. This itself goes a long way toward making for a reasonable result. Free conditions for citizen input helps to assure that the conclusions of public debate will themselves be reached freely since coercion, bribery, and all forms of intimidation will have to be prohibited. Democracy, of course, has its flaws; the whole of society or any democratically organized part of it may become irrational, jealous of individual excellence, or fixed in its narrow self-interest. But as dangerous as these possibilities are, they mirror directly the very same dangers inherent in defending personal autonomy, since persons, too, can become irrational, threatened by the excellence of others, and narrowly self-interested. Our hope in the case of persons is that continuous and vigorous use of personal autonomy will tend to override these dangers and will tend to build persons with feelings and habits more and more well suited to free and rational choosing. A similar hope animates our embrace of democracy. The society structured around democratic social habits will tend to produce autonomous persons who have feelings and habits increasingly and spontaneously well suited to free and rational social choosing.

Democracy can take two different expressions, both of which are important for our concerns.[1] First, attaining practical social autonomy means institutionalizing political democracy. This is first in importance because the political institutions of a society control the consolidated force and power of that society and determine its uses. Thus political democracy sets the factual horizon for all other democratic experiences by assuring that the consolidated force and power of a society aids and does not inhibit further democratic social expressions. Political democracy itself has two necessary components. There must be equal access of all citizens to influence on and control of political authority. This component may take many creative expressions but the most obvious one is a political system of universal adult suffrage where each adult person's vote counts equally with all others. The second necessary component of political democracy is the construction of a system for the political protection of persons' equal moral rights. The most obvious way to institutionalize this element is through specification of these moral rights as legal rights and through provision of mechanisms for judicial enforcement of these legal rights.[2] Thus political democracy can be viewed as the social expression of our duty to recognize and respect the equal rights of all persons by creating equal access to the consolidated power of society and equal legal rights before an impartial legal system.

When our political duties are thus discharged, the building of democratic habits in all of society's remaining institutions and practices is an important means of building practical social autonomy.[3] The real ability of persons to participate meaningfully in the shaping of the social facts of their lives can enrich and deepen the significance of their practical personal autonomies by helping to draw together the private and social dimensions of their lives in the context of free and rational choice. The private self and the social self can be drawn together by personal participation in social realities. Thus, personal autonomy may be directly enhanced by the building of democratic habits of free and full participation in families, schools, churches, local communities, workplaces, and wherever social institutions and practices significantly shape persons' lives. Since we are dealing here with values beyond duty, there will be a rich creative element in the democratic restructuring of social institutions, a creative element which must respond to tradition; idiosyncrasies of person, time, and place; and the demands of other important social values. In spite of this inevitable variety, there is a central core to democratic social habits and to the nature of a progressive society: the free and equal participation of persons in the shaping and control of the social settings which shape and control their individual lives. Thus democracy at the social level is an important means of protecting, enhancing, and maximizing practical personal autonomy.

One of the most critical institutions in contemporary society is the modern hospital. Hospitals and the hospital experience have undergone dramatic changes in this century, changes which make the achievement of democratic social habits here of unique human importance. If we want hospitals to be an aid and not a hinderance to the growth of social autonomy and the growth in personal autonomy which this entails, then we must set as a goal the democratization of the hospital. Before we specify the nature and direction of this democratization, it is important to state explicitly the reasons why the hospital has now become an appropriate institution for such attention.

The modern hospital is now an unavoidable institution.[4] Most of us are now born in hospitals and most of us die there. Many of life's most critical turning points between birth and death occur there as well, especially the major operations which save and reshape our lives. This was not always so. The vast majority of persons throughout human history have been born and have died at home and have been without the benefits of the major medical interventions between birth and death which we now take for granted. The twentieth century hospital is thus a powerful new social fact. Regardless of how sick or well we are just now, the chances are very good that each of us will spend a significant amount of time in a hospital.

When we turn to hospitals, we generally do so with an overriding sense of need for the services there. Generally, this is when we are experiencing pain, suffering, loss of practical personal autonomy, or the fixated negative self-consciousness of the sick. Often we are medically helpless without the hospital; sometimes in peril for our lives. At times, the lives of those we love are turned over wholly to the care of the hospital. And hospital patients are not good consumers for reasons we have already indicated. All of this adds up to a substantial vulnerability on the part of hospital patients before the institutional power of the modern hospital.

It is also evident now that the running of the modern hospital is a big business.[5] As such, today's hospital is subject to the pressures of the market, investors and contributors, and of the accepted cost cutting and price setting mechanisms of the business world. If the bureaucratic management of the contemporary hospital is not evidence enough of this significant business dimension, surely a contemporary hospital bill is.

The specialization and subspecialization of today's medicine and the division of labor expressing the general demands of economic efficiency have resulted in a marked fragmentation of care in the hospital. The typical hospital patient has a difficult time identifying the names and tasks of the various health care professionals who trail in and out of the hospital room. Not only can this fragmentation of care be emotionally and financially unsettling to the patient, but it can also dilute the authority a patient has over his or her care. The confusions generated by such a situation can factually diminish a patient's ability to understand and consent.

Finally, the modern hospital experience is one of the most direct and intimate encounters the average person has with the new powers of science and technology.[6] Of course, each of us is immersed in a world replete with scientific and technological powers. Yet seldom does this power appear to be exercised directly for us. In the hospital, the full weight of our modern knowledge and technique is applied for the benefit of the individual person. Thus, the hospital experience for most people is a formative encounter with the contemporary world. Science and technology, because of their inherent difficulty and distance from direct impact on daily life, contain a decided tendency toward elitism. The modern hospital patient is in the hands of a would-be scientific and technical elite and is reminded so constantly by the specialized language and jargon which they share but which the patient does not. The character of this hospital experience will help to form the general attitude of persons in our society towards science, technology, and the apparent elite who know and operate these tools. The future will bring even more power to science and technology and will exacerbate this tendency toward elitism. Part of the response a democratic society will make to this challenge is being shaped in the habits embedded in today's hospital.

For these reasons we must seek to build habits leading to social autonomy in the hospital; we must strive to democratize the hospital experience. In the first place, the political expression of this demand will issue in a concern for the specification and enforcement of the moral rights of hospital patients as legal rights. Secondly, the social expression of this demand will lead us to seek to maximize the attainment of practical personal autonomy in the hospital through fuller and freer participation by all those involved. These are not unrelated tasks. The building of institutionalized habits of political democracy serves to protect our practical personal autonomy, as the building of democratic habits in all social institutions and practices serves to enhance the factual development and enjoyment of that autonomy. There is no escaping the fact that we will continue to institutionalize our medical care. The moral question which faces us is whether or not this institutionalization will embody our moral ideals as well. If our ethical theory demands that we everywhere seek to maximize practical person autonomy, then we must seek ways of doing this within the social habits of the modern hospital as well.

B. Legal Rights in the Hospital

Preserving and accelerating the advance of political democracy as it bears on the contemporary hospital, requires that we acknowledge and respect hospital patients' rights. Many of the ideal moral rights of hospital patients have entered the factual arena of legal rights. Thus they have acquired a reality assured by the implied force consolidated in our political institutions in our courts, legislatures, and police departments. Compared therefore to the task of determining the moral rights of a person, determining a person's legal rights is a more straightforward enterprise. But even here caution must be expressed at the outset because considerable intepretation is still necessary when dealing with court decisions, state and federal legislation, and the separate but at times ovelapping jurisdictions of state and federal law. With this caution, the following appear to be some of the most significant legal rights of hospital patients.[7]

Let us begin theoretically where many of us in fact begin our encounter with the hospital, in the emergency room. Most U.S. courts recognize a person's right to emergency treatment if a true emergency exists and the hospital has made its emergency facilities publicly known and publicly available. The trend in the law is toward holding the hospital responsible for providing emergency care to the public when the public has come to rely on the availability of such care. Referral by or approval of one's own physician for needed emergency care is legally irrelevant to this right of access. In **Wilmington General Hospital v. Manlove**, the Delaware Supreme Court held a hospital negligent for refusing to treat an infant (who subsequently died) because the emergency room nurse could not contact the child's physician. The Court wrote, ". . . that liability on the part of a hospital may be predicated on the refusal of service to a patient in case of an unmistakeable emergency, if the patient has relied upon a well-established custom of the hospital to render aid in such a case."[8]

This right of access to needed emergency care cannot be qualified by ability to pay. In a bona fide emergency, a person has a right to treatment at a hospital on whose emergency care the public has come to rely whether or not that person can demonstrate ability to pay. The Wisconsin Supreme Court has written: "It would shock the public conscience if a person in need of emergency aid would be turned down at the door of a hospital having emergency service because the person could not at that moment assure payment for the service."[9] An Arizona Supreme Court ruling has extended this legal right even further, when it ruled that a person has a legal right of access to emergency care regardless of ability to pay and regardless of that person's status as a nonresident alien.[10] These decisions imply that the legal right to emergency care cannot be qualified by money or citizenship.

There is no clear legal right to subsequent admission to the hospital for nonemergency care. Hospitals, and especially private hospitals, have the legal right to refuse patients, to screen those who seek admission, and to require a down payment or evidence of health insurance. On the other hand, patients have the right not to be denied hospital admission on the discriminatory bases of race, color, national origin, or residency requirements.

Presuming that he or she has successfully gained admission to some hospital, today's patient has a legally recognized right to informed consent. Since Judge Cardozo's opinion in **Schloendorff v. Society of New York Hospital**, courts have recognized this doctrine of informed consent and based it on the principle that "(e)very human being of adult years and sound mind has a right to determine what shall be done with his own body . . . ."[11] Thus, freedom from medical coercions is protected by law. Of course, this right to bodily self-determination cannot be meaningfully exercised without the information needed to make reasonable decisions. Therefore, the legal doctrine of informed consent imposes a duty on the physician to explain proposed medical procedures to the patient and to warn of any material risks inherent in or collateral to the proposed therapy. This legal duty on the part of the physician enables the patient to exercise the legal right to make a free and informed choice about whether or not to undergo such treatment.[12] Only two exceptions to this rule have surfaced in court decisions. The right to be informed is suspended if the patient is unconscious or if the risk of disclosure poses such a threat of detriment to the patient as to become contraindicated from a medical point of view.[13]

While courts are in general agreement on the principle of informed consent, there is some significant disagreement about the scope of the physician's duty to warn. Since the average patient has considerably less medical and scientific knowledge than the physician, some legal standard must be employed to determine just how much of the physician's knowledge of procedures and risks must be conveyed to the patient. There appears to be two legal options here. Some courts have adhered to a professional standard of informed consent under which the degree of the physician's obligation to disclose is a matter of professional judgment based on what is usually disclosed by competent physicians in similar cases.[14] Courts employing such a standard require expert medical testimony to determine from within the medical profession itself the customary degree of disclosure. However, other courts have focused on the informational needs of the individual patient and found that the appropriate test is not what is customary for physicians but what is reasonable conduct under the circumstances. Since what is reasonable may be judged independently of what is professionally customary, this test of the degree of information provided by the physician is a lay person's standard. This lay standard of informed consent has been expressed as a materiality test whereby the scope of the physician's disclosure duty is measured by the materiality or importance of the information to the decision-making of the patient. Thus, on this interpretation, the degree of information to be provided is measured by what is reasonable given the particular choice needs of the patient.[15]

The legal situation is further complicated by state legislation. Between 1975 and 1977, twenty-four states enacted legislation dealing with informed consent in response to the so-called medical malpractice crisis of 1974-76. Though these laws have made many minor changes, they do not seem to have substantially altered the general legal nature of the informed consent doctrine. So, while it is advisable for a hospital patient to be aware of the judicial test for the scope of the legal right to informed consent and the pertinent state legislation in the jurisdiction, a hospital patient does have a legal right to be free from subjection to any hospital procedure without his or her voluntary and understanding consent.

129

A hospital patient also some legal rights with respect to hospital records. Access to such records can be an important ingredient in the composition of an informed consent since these records may contain information relevant to the making of reasonable choices. On the other hand, in a position analogous to the professional standard of informed consent, the American Medical Association has held that the patient's physician should decide if and how much of a patient's records should be made available.[16] If the physician should refuse to cooperate, a few states allow direct patient access to records, but most states allow for access only by subpoena in the event of a lawsuit against the hospital or physician. The legal difficulty from a patient's point of view is that the hospital has physical possession of records, and these documents are the hospital's property. Although one court has held that a patient does have a property right in the information contained in the records and thus may not be denied access to them, another court has ruled that a former mental patient who sought to obtain hospital records for the purposes of writing a book had no constitutionally protected right to inspect or copy her own records.[17]

If a patient should ever want access to other hospital patients' records in a malpractice suit, the hospital or physician will likely resist such access on the grounds that the professional privilege of confidentially protects both hospital and physician from the obligation of disclosing these files. The trend in the courts seems to be to order disclosure of other patients' records in a lawsuit so long as the patients' identities are protected.[18] Furthermore, a patient has very little legal protection against the disclosure of his or her records to others. Though a physician's direct communication with a patient has traditionally been regarded as privileged, the legal implications of this tradition are not clear: As yet no patient has ever recovered damages from a doctor due to an alleged breach of confidentiality.[19] Consequently, it is legally unclear what binding responsibility a physician has with respect to patients' hospital records. The hospital as custodian of the records may itself have no duty of confidentiality to the patients whose records they hold. Moreover, many hospitals are joining information pools and storing their medical records with centralized computer systems. This trend may make it even more difficult to assure privacy of hospital patients' records. In summary, a patient may have no legal right of access to his or her own hospital records unless a lawsuit against the hospital or physician is initiated, and at present a patient may have very little legal control over who else does have access to them.

The legal right of informed consent, of course, guarantees by implication the general right to refuse any medical therapy. The reasons given for such refusal may even be irrelevant. One commentator on the law has argued that a patient has an absolute right to refuse medical treatment for whatever reason.[20] The courts, however, are in disagreement about a patient's right to refuse treatment in life threatening situations where refusal will bring on an otherwise preventable death. In one series of cases dealing with Jehovah's Witnesses who refused lifesaving blood transfusions, the courts appointed guardians with authority to consent to the transfusions in spite of the patients' refusals. These decisions were justified by the claim that the state's interest in maintaining life supercedes the individual's religious beliefs.[21] However, in an Illinois Supreme Court decision, **In re Estate of Brooks**, the court reversed a lower court's order which had appointed a conservator or guardian to authorize the transfusion for a refusing Jehovah's Witness.[22] This court found "no clear and present danger" warranting interference with the patient's religious proscriptions. Thus, while it appears that in most cases a patient has the legal right to refuse any medical treatment, this right may be overturned in the case of needed lifesaving treatments, at least in cases involving procedures deemed to be medically ordinary and in situations where death is neither inevitable nor proximate.

If a patient is facing a terminal illness, the right to refuse aggressive death prolonging treatment is protected by the constitutionally implied right to privacy.[23] Recent cases dealing with a patient's right to refuse treatment in terminal situations have centered around the related problem of incompetent patients: whether or not the courts can allow a competent third party to assert an incompetent patient's right to refuse. In the case of Karen Quinlan, the court concluded that her privacy right would permit the refusal of further treatment and that this constitutional protection could be asserted for her by her parent. In **Superintendent v. Saikewicz**, the Supreme Judicial Court of Massachusetts held that in situations where medical personnel must decide whether an incompetent and terminally ill patient should receive further aggressive treatment, the personnel must petition the court for the appointment of a guardian and the judge must conduct a hearing on whether the treatment should be provided.[24] In both cases, then, courts have allowed a means for a competent third party to assert an incompetent terminal patient's right to refuse further aggressive measures to sustain life. In a third important case in this area, **Custody of a Minor**, a court denied the alleged right of a minor's parents to refuse lifesaving chemotherapy for him.[25] In this case, the Massachusetts Supreme Judicial Court affirmed a lower court's order awarding custody of the child to the state so that he could be given therapy over his parents' objections. The court here relied on the doctrine of substituted judgment as outlined in the **Saikewicz** case and a traditional "best interest of the child" test. It seems to follow from these cases that even if a patient should become incompetent, his or her right to accept or reject treatments can be exercised by some third party, though at this time there is disagreement in the legal community as to who that third party should be.

Finally, a hospital patient has both the legal right not to be discharged from the hospital prematurely and the legal right to leave the hospital at any time regardless of whether medical treatment is deemed complete. Premature discharge or discharge against a patient's will may constitute medical abandonment and hospital patients have the legal right not to be abandoned.[26] As we have already seen, once the doctor-patient relationship has commenced, the law requires that it continue until it is ended by the parties' mutual consent, it is revoked by the patient, the physician's services are no longer needed, or the physician withdraws from the case after reasonable notice to the patient. Abandonment of a patient outside of these conditions may result in a malpractice action against the doctor, although unreasonable demands or lack of cooperation by the patient may be considered the legal equivalent of revocation of the relationship by the patient. On the other hand, a competent patient may leave the hospital at any time he or she chooses even if treatment is incomplete and even if the hospital bill has not been paid.[27] If the hospital should try to prevent a competent patient from leaving, the hospital may be sued by the patient for false imprisonment, i.e., intentional and wrongful confinement by another against one's will.[28]

These are some of the most important legal rights of hospital patients. They represent the furthest advance which the ideal of human autonomy has made in fact in our legal system in this context. They embody certain clear achievements. But from our autonomy maximization perspective they just as clearly leave much to be done if we are to legally protect practical personal autonomy in the hospital. We can tend to the unfinished business, or some of it, now.

C. Hospital Democracy

In many cases, the distinction between those rights which we are bond to respect from duty and those values whose attainment is morally regulative but not strictly obligatory; in many cases, this distinction is not precise. In other terms, there is often an overlap or a shading between what is done to protect human autonomy and what is done to enhance it. Political democracy issues in legal rights which we are duty bound to recognize. Social democracy opens new possibilities for the enhancement of practical personal autonomy through the free participation of persons in the shaping of those dimensions of life that shape them in turn. Intermediate between these concerns are moral rights, rights which issue from our concern to protect human dignity but which are not codified as law in fact. These moral rights often point to substantial enhancements of human autonomy by the isolation of values we should seek to maximize. Before moving directly to a consideration of the democratization of the hospital experience let us consider three moral rights which fulfill the duty to protect practical personal autonomy to a fuller extent than that now mandated by law and which point the way to additional enhancements of that autonomy.

As we have seen, the Wisconsin Supreme Court found that denying emergency care to those unable to pay for it would "shock the public conscience." We may well be approaching the day when our emotions will have been so infused with the ideals we have embraced that the denial of hospital admission to any indigent person in true need of nonemergency care will shock the public conscience as well. The very affluence of our society, the ubiquity of hospitals, and the massive public investment already made to foster medical education, research, and the delivery of health care make it appropriate and factually possible to now demand what is morally ideal: a moral right for all persons to gain admission to some hospital for necessary nonemergency medical care regardless of ability to pay. Such a moral right will have to be specified practically. There is probably no natural limit to what medical services may be made available in the future, and the moral right at issue here cannot be meant to assert a claim of such inexhaustible nature. Instead, some reasonable minimum standard of health care should be defined (and redefined as our technology and ideals develop) and made available to all persons in our society regardless of ability to pay.

Of course, to acknowledge a right to hospital admission is virtually to admit a right to health care itself. This is a highly emotional political issue, the many dimensions of which cannot be sorted out here, but some observations are in order nonetheless.[29] Since 1948, the United States has been committed to the United Nations' "Universal Declaration of Human Rights" (the same document the Soviet bloc accepted at Helsinki in 1975). Article 25(1) of that statement reads: "Everyone has the right to a standard of living adequate for the health and well-being of himself and his family, including food, clothing, housing, and medical care and necessary social services. . . ."[30] Whether the various assistance programs now in place (Medicare, Medicaid, etc.) are sufficient to satisfy the intent of this acknowledged moral right is highly debatable. In any event, the United States is the only industrialized nation in the world today without a system of governmentally paid health services for all its citizens.[31] It would seem to be incompatible with the achievement of maximal practical personal autonomy that some persons go without adequate health care because of their inability to pay for it. The demand for health care arises out of an overriding and unequally distributed need. From a moral perspective, these needs, and not money, are the critical consideration in answering that demand.[32] Moreover, acknowledging a moral right to health care would be an important way to concretely assert the incalculably great value which each person is to the human community. Thus, a right to be admitted to some hospital ought to be guaranteed, whether satisfaction of that right takes the shape of a more adequate version of the present United States' system, national health insurance, or a national health care service.

A second moral right we should assert for persons once they become hospital patients is the right to a lay standard for measuring the degree of information mandated by the doctrine of informed consent, not merely the customary standards of professional medicine. Professional customs, in medicine as in all professions, can be self-serving or blind habits and are therefore in need of public scrutiny. More importantly, the moral point of the doctrine of informed consent is to provide the patient with the rational wherewithal to make an intelligent choice, as such the criterion of the adequacy of the information provided must make direct reference to the patient's choice needs. And, as we have already seen, there is evidence to suggest that the doctor-patient relationship is more medically effective when the sort of communicative openness and sharing called for by the doctrine of informed consent prevails. Patient centered information sharing is critical for the development of these relationships of mutual participation. Therefore, we ought to recognize patients' moral right to informed consent and insist that the medical information provided to them include all the facts and options which could have a material effect on their decision-making.

Finally, we should recognize a moral right of access to one's own hospital records. Information can be a powerful means of exploitation or personal growth. The collection of hospital records in central computer banks raises far-reaching moral questions about control by others over a person's own life. If the information contained in these computers is false, damaging, or just plain unpopular and it reaches the wrong hands, a former hospital patient may lose jobs, promotions, insurance, etc., quite beyond his or her own control. This is unfair and a compromise of practical personal autonomy. Unless ways are found to guarantee the confidentiality of such computer stored information, patients ought to be able to see precisely what is in their hospital records so they can prevent unfair damage to themselves. At the same time, access to hospital records can be an important educational tool for one's return to wellness and for preventive medical care. Of course, these records can be misunderstood by poorly educated patients, but this possibility itself can present an opportunity for further medical teaching and learning. Though the actual pieces of paper or microfilm of patients' records may legally be the property of the hospital, patients ought to have the moral right to see them, to understand them, and to grow in rational self-control through them.

Recognition of these moral rights would help to complete the protection of the law and point in the direction of greater participation by persons in the hospital, in this institution which can so intimately shapes our lives. Guaranteeing access to the hospital itself means that all persons in our society, regardless of financial situation, will have access to participation in the great benefits of contemporary hospital care. Guaranteeing communication in laymen's terms and about risks that are materially significant from a patient's point of view means that all patients will have an opportunity to meaningful exercise their right to informed consent, and will thus be able to participate in decision-making relevant to their own care. Guaranteeing access to hospital records means that patients will be able to participate in the composition and storage of intimate information about themselves and will be able to more completely understand their conditions.

Additional participation by hospital patients can be achieved in ways which go beyond duty toward the attainment of values inherent in our commitment to maximizing practical personal autonomy. First, hospital patients should be routinely informed of their legal rights. Measures should be taken to insure that each hospital patient is made aware of the legal rights we have described. A copy of a statement of hospital patient rights should be distributed to each patient on admission to the hospital or should be posted plainly in each hospital room. Furthermore, every hospital should have a patient rights' advocate or ombudsman whose job it should be to insure that patients know their legal rights and how to initiate complaints if and when those rights are violated. Such a person might have to be in the employ of a group or institution other than the hospital itself to avoid the obvious conflict of interest here.

However the specifics of such an arrangement are worked out, the main issue here is that the unavoidability of the hospital, the overriding need for its services, the big business aspects of hospital care, the fragmentation of hospital care, and the contact with a powerful science and technology in the hands of a hospital elite all conspire to make the hospital patient highly vulnerable. Protection of such vulnerability requires legal rights, but such rights become practically meaningless for most hospital patients if their existence and purpose is not made clear. Recall here the negative and fixated consciousness of the sick. A stay in the hospital is not the time when most of us are willing, able, or even interested in asserting our rights. A society which seeks to maximize practical personal autonomy will guarantee that hospital patients know of these legal rights and are aided and encouraged to exercise them.

Second, efforts should be made to involve patients directly in the day to day affairs of hospital life. Obviously, some patients are incapable of any meaningful contribution to hospital life. But when hospital patients are able to, they should be given some voice on such nonmedical aspects of their care as meals, visiting hours, room assignments, access to television and radio, etc. Patients should have periodic meetings to discuss these and any other issues of importance to them. There should be patient councils for the entire hospital. These points may seem trivial or potential sources of confusion, but it must be remembered that hospital patients are autonomous persons. They are not prisoners. Increased control over any parts of life, even over when a snack bar is available or when newspapers are distributed, can help restore a measure of the practical personal autonomy which is sacrificed when sickness forces a stay in the hospital. Even if some confusion does result from these measures, they may be well worth the price if, as our earlier discussion of mutual participation suggests, there is a therapeutic value to participation with one's care. In any event, some confusion is such a sure sign of real personal and social autonomy that it ought never to be shied away from on its own account. Confusion often initiates a rethinking of presumptions, a rethinking that can lead to creative innovation and progress.

Third, because hospital patients are so often incapable of such participation by virtue of their sickness or because of the brevity of their stays in the hospital, some other group directly and keenly interested in patient welfare should be involved in the shaping of hospital habits. Every hospital should have a community appointed board of citizens or of recent patients which would meet to review patient complaints of rights violations and to propose measures to further enhance the human quality of the hospital experience.

One more suggestion may be useful here. Those health care professionals most directly concerned for hospital patients' welfare on a day to day professional basis are hospital nurses. One cannot help but think that patient care would be improved generally and practical personal autonomy enhanced if nurses had greater authority in the structuring and restructuring of social habits in the modern hospital. The modern nurse has a medical education second only to the physician's, and unlike the physician, the hospital nurse deals with the total needs of the hospital patient, twenty four hours a day. It is the nurse who knows first and most surely when a hospital patient's rights have been or are about to be violated. It is the nurse who is best disposed to see what practical measure should be taken to enhance the care and increase the practical personal autonomy of patients. Nurses are well placed to reintegrate fragmented hospital care and to see to it that a patient's encounter with science, technology, and the elites that run them in the hospital is a humanly satisfying one. Furthermore, increased democratic control of hospitals by the nursing staff would go a long way toward establishing nurses' collective autonomy over the working conditions that daily shape their own lives. Such an increase in control and authority by hospital nurses would thus create a sphere of relative professional autonomy and help diminish some of the professional alienation now felt by hospital nurses.[33]

These measures and others like them can take us beyond duty to the attainment of other human values in the contemporary hospital. In the hospital, we institutionalize our care and cure of one another, and as we do we build social habits by which we define ourselves and our society. If the hospital is a place of patient servility and deference to a medical and bureaucratic elite, then the hospital experience will tend to build persons who are subservient and deferential and will help prepare the ground for the general loss of our social and personal freedoms. If the hospital is a place of respect for patient equality and autonomy, then the hospital experience will tend to build persons who are equal and autonomous and will help preserve and enhance all our social and personal freedoms. If we are to truly embrace the ideals of autonomous persons in progressive societies, we must work to democratize the modern hospital so as to maximize practical personal autonomy in the human experiences which occur between its walls.

Chapter 11.

Medical Research

A. Using Human Subjects In Research

If the hospital sets the social context for the present delivery of medical care, this is only possible because of a significant social dimension of medicine's past: medical research. There are two clear social elements here. First is the fact that like science itself, medical science has advanced because an historically self-conscious group of researchers has bound itself to habits of methodical, even tedious, examination of the human body and its relationship to its environment, and because these researchers have accumulated and passed on the information thereby gained as a social property. Information about the causes, prevention, and treatment of sickness and, more recently, information on the means to promote wellness has been selflessly collected, organized, and made available for the benefit of an indefinitely large number of persons in the present and into the future. There is probably no finer example of the ability of human persons to transcend the limitations of time, place, and national, racial, and ideological differences for the sake of serving humanity. In this manner, the great benefits of modern medicine have come to us as a collective inheritance.

The second clearly social element of medical research, and the one which will be pursued here since it raises important moral issues, is the fact that much of this medical research has been conducted with the use of human persons as subjects. The drugs which cure us today were first tried experimentally on other persons. The routine surgery done everywhere today was first done experimentally on some other persons. The drugs not used today and the surgeries not done today because in both cases they were found to be unsafe, were found to be so after they were tried experimentally on some persons. Most of these persons are impossible to name; perhaps some did not even know they were experimental subjects. In any case, we and those who follow us in the future owe these individual persons of the past a great debt. Our health care is the powerful armamentarium it is today in large part because of the sacrifices of these few.

If medicine is to continue to increase and perfect its abilities to care for persons who are sick and to cure their diseases, research using human subjects will have to continue in the present and into the foreseeable future. Without continued use of human subjects in medical research, either no new drugs, surgeries, or other medical techniques will become publicly available. If they do become available without being tested on humans, then the first group of persons receiving these therapies clinically will be experimental subjects **de facto**. Either there will be no medical innovations, or there will be medical research with human subjects who are not aware that they are research subjects. When persons are not aware of being used as subjects, the research they are involved in will likely be unacceptable both scientifically and morally since the full range of experimental controls will be lacking, as will the honesty which respect for the rights of the subjects demands. Continued medical advance, therefore, requires the mutually self-conscious use of human persons as research subjects. Laboratory and animals studies should be used to minimize the use of human subjects, of course, but in the final analysis, there is no scientifically nor morally acceptable alternative to the testing of new medical techniques experimentally on human subjects before these techniques are brought into general clinical use. The only real alternative is to stop the progress of medicine altogether. The moral unacceptability of this alternative is clear in a moment if one considers the increase in human suffering and earlier deaths and the decrease in practical personal antonomy we should have to live with today had such a cessation in medical research occurred a decade ago or a century ago. Clearly, there is a strong moral imperative to continue the advance of medical science, an imperative coextensive with the duty and desire to care for and cure the sick.

There is a wide range of medical experimentation with humans which involves no appreciable risk to the subjects; for example, routine acquisition of height and weight information for statistical research, collection and examination of human excreta, and experimental regulation of foods normally in the diet. Subjects in such experiments face no more danger than that normally associated with daily living itself. While some other important moral considerations are pertinent even here, moral issues related to risk are not. On the other hand, many medical experiments involve the giving of a new drug or the performance of a novel procedure. Typically, the subject's reaction to the drug or procedure is carefully monitored, records made regarding the whole exchange, and the information stored and eventually made available to the medical profession at large. If such an experiment is to have a reasonable scientific goal, then the effect of the drug or procedure on humans must be little understood in general, or if the general effects be known, the specific quantities or details for specific purposes little understood. In short, if something is to be learned, it must be because something is not known or not securely known. It is this very ignorance which makes research necessary and which constitutes the danger to the research subject. Consequently, in all such experiments, there must be some degree of risk to the subject.

Imposing a risk on a human being for the benefit of other human beings appears, at least initially, to be straightforwardly incompatible with the incalculably great value we have attributed to each individual person. This becomes plain if the context of experimentation is changed even slightly. Suppose a nonscientist and nonphysician were to set out to test the reaction of persons to various drugs and procedures out of pure personal curiosity, caprice, or malice. Without the justification of possible medical progress, the giving of a new drug to a person or the use of some novel bodily procedure on a human person would be morally outrageous. It seems too clearly an assault on human autonomy, too clearly a use of a person as a thing for some other purpose or benefit. But the addition of the medical research context and the medical progress it seeks certainly adds a significant dimension to our moral intuitions here. If medical care is a value, then the experimentation needed to continually enhance that care is a value as well. The context of possible medical progress embeds medical research within a larger value commitment; and not just any value commitment, but a strong and traditional one, the fruits of which have benefited and will continue to benefit an indefinitely large number of other persons in the present and into the future.

In order to adjudicate this tension in our moral intuitions, let us recall that the central focus of our absolute valuation of every human person is the value creative activity of each self. This value creative activity is the ability of the practically autonomous person to freely and rationally take a person, object, or activity up into his or her world as a value. The self as source of this valuing ability then is the value of values. Consequently, no other value can be so compelling that it can be used to justify an assault on the person's incalculably valuable self. On this account, even the use of one person for the sake of benefit to several other persons is unacceptable, since two or more incalculably great values are no more valuable together than one is alone, just as two or more infinities is still equal to infinity. On the other hand, it is just because the self of the person can so freely embrace other values that the self is the creator of, and thus value of, values. This insight provides for the possibility of an ethical resolution to our moral confusion on the acceptability of medical research on human subjects. Because of our conception of the individual person's value, the attainment of no other value, including the progress of medicine and its ability to aid innumerable other persons, is sufficient grounds for forcing or deceiving a human person into a medical experiment. But at the same time, since our valuation of the person turns on the self's ability to embrace other values, the free and understanding choice by a person to become an experimental subject is morally acceptable. Indeed, since the practically autonomous assumption of such a risk is a self-sacrifice critically important to the lives and wellness of other persons and is also a contribution potentially satisfying to the research subject too, a free choice of this nature is a noble act which ought to be individually praised and collectively encouraged through our personal and social habits.

It follows then that the informed consent of the subject is a necessary condition for the moral acceptability of the use of human persons in medical experimentation. This moral demand for the free and understanding choice of the subject before participation in a medical experiment rules out any justification for the use of persons who have not given such consent. Specifically, this means that regardless of the perceived benefits to others in particular or to society in general, the initiation of experimental risk against a person's will or without their knowledge is morally unacceptable. Though this rejection of a risk-benefit calculation shares much in common with our earlier rejection of happiness maximizing utilitarianism, the reasons in this context for the rejection of such calculations must be made explicit because the attractiveness of the value of aiding in the advance of medical progress is so strong that it can blind medical researchers and their professional associates to the other moral values and duties at stake.

First, if a human person is an incalcublably great value, then a person cannot be assigned a cardinal number value, nor can one human person be ordinally ranked before or after another in value. All human persons are of equal value because all are of an indefinitely great value. It makes no moral sense, therefore, to place one person at risk to benefit two, since two persons are no more valuable together than one is alone. As human dignity transcends price, it cannot be computed, exchanged, replaced, or made equivalent to another value. Thus, while it may be quite reasonable, for example, to kill and dissect one cow to prevent disease from spreading through a whole herd of twenty cows, such a risk-benefit calculation is absolutely incompatible with the dignity and consequent rights of a human person. By comparison to the obligatory value of each human person, the worthy cause of medical progress is an optional value. If aiding the cause of medical progress is an optional value, it can only be served if the persons involved, the obligatory values, truely and knowingly opt to participate. This entails the conclusion we have already drawn: All participation by human subjects in medical experiments must be voluntary. No person may be forced or deceived into taking a risk for the benefit of others. This is so regardless of the alleged social uselessness of the subject of the experiment or the magnitude of the expected benefit to others.

Secondly, were we to adopt such risk-benefit reasoning, we could justify the use of human subjects for virtually any experiment with a reasonable scientific purpose. There are always persons in every society who are deemed less important by social convention and therefore less of a risk to lose or to harm. At the same time, the number of those persons benefited in the future by the medical progress made possible by these losses and harms can always be calculated to be indefinitely large, and these beneficiaries will surely include persons thought to be more socially worthy than the subjects who are used. We might, for example, count every child born after the discovery of some vaccination against a severe childhood disease as a beneficiary of this discovery. Surely this massive group contains innumerable geniuses of all sorts. Suppose now that in the early stages of experiment with this vaccine, it is proposed that it be tested without consent of any sort on terminally ill and mentally handicapped children. From the perspective of a risk-benefit calculation, this appears to be an irresistibly good bargain: All children into the indefinite future benefit while the risks are contained to those who are already impaired and near death. But from the ethical perspective we have assumed, this is plainly unacceptable. Informed consent, in this case that of parent or guardian, is an absolutely necessary precondition for such a test (though it may not be sufficient, in light of what will be said later). A straightforward calculation of risks and benefits then, without reference to the incalculably great value of each human person, can and likely will lead to such unethical and intuitively immoral results.

Thirdly, the assignment of the relative values needed for a risk-benefit calculation is not susceptible to any objective testing whatsoever. What numbers, for example, do we assign to each vaccinated child and what numbers to the incompetent and dying children on whom the vaccine is tested? In such a situation, numerical gradings of risks and benefits must be considered morally arbitrary. Given such wholesale arbitrariness, self-serving assumptions will inevitably arise. The estimate of risks to unpopular or inarticulate groups will likely be depressed; estimate of benefits to favored and vocal groups will likely be inflated. Moreover, the whole calculative process is subject to the self-interest of the researcher and the self-interests built into our entire health care system. It would be more than naive not to admit the mixture of motives in any human enterprise, medical science included. Reputation, promotion, and financial reward are as influential in the medical scientist's life as they are in the lives of businessmen, politicians, and philosophers. When the numbering of human risk and benefit has no objective basis, these factors will surely come more prominently into play in the experimental context. It would be equally naive not to recognize the impact of the profit motivation of much of the contemporary health care industry. Unbridled risk-benefit calculation in such an environment will certainly be skewed, however unconsciously, to serve the interests of investors, hospitals, and those who produce and sell the drugs and technologies on which modern medicine depends.

Finally, a simple calculation of risks and benefits is likely to overlook the intangible risks to science and medicine generally should the public begin to believe that they are being exploited in experimental contexts. The social trust necessary to attract public and private funds for medical research and to elicit volunteers for needed medical experimentation is a fragile value, risks to which, though real, are subtle and hard to measure. Such calculation is also likely to underrate the intangible benefits to society from the very existence of a scientifically competent and medically humane research community which graphically expresses our moral ideals by refusing to advance itself at the cost of harms to human persons. Who can measure the indefinitely great moral benefits to society from the example of such a collective commitment?

One general rule of ethics here as elsewhere is that we can seek attainment of other important human values only after our duty to respect persons has been discharged. We can seek to advance medical science and thus aid in the effort to promote an increase in human pleasure, happiness, and practical personal autonomy by decreasing human sickness, promoting better medical care, and extending human life, but only if the rights of all persons are respected in the process. Assuring that we always have the voluntary and understanding consent of subjects in medical arch allows us to seek to achieve these important values and to do our ⌐ to others. There is a dynamic and compelling attractiveness to the idea of medical progress, but such progress, as valuable as it is, will not be worth having if we lose respect for the source of all values along the way. Risk-benefit calculations may indeed hasten medical progress and the attainment of the important values associated with that progress, but if the considerations presented here are accurate, it will do so at a morally unacceptable cost.[1] In terms of moral importance, our duty to the individual human person precedes the value of all forms of human progress because without that obligatory value, no other value can be a value at all.

B. Abuses and Vulnerabilities

The potential for the exploitation of persons in the service of medical research is not only a theoretical possibility in the ideal, it is also an historical fact of not so long ago and not so far away. For examples of such abuses, consider the following experiments which have all been conducted since the end of World War II by American researchers.[2] It is a reasonable supposition that this record of known abuses represents only a fraction of similar but unknown abuses.

Children have been exploited in some cases. For instance, to test whether or not urethal reflux can occur in normal bladders, vesicourethrography was carried out on 26 normal babies less than forty-eight hours old. These infants were then exposed to x-rays while their bladders were filling and voiding. Even children seeking medical aid have been used. Of 130 children being studied to record the effect of hyposensitization therapy for bronchial asthma, 91 received therapeutically inert injections of buffered saline for periods of up to 14 years without the knowledge of either child or parent.

Prisoners have been subjected to much abuse. Prisoners in Oregon submitted to repeated bilateral testicular biopsies and injections of radioactive thymidine to test the rate of spermatogenesis. In California, extreme "acting-out" criminal offenders were involved in aversive conditioning experiments with a drug that creates muscle paralysis and sensations of suffocation. Five of these prisoners later claimed they had been forced to participate against their wills and eighteen reported that they had felt pressured. Eleven prisoners in Iowa submitted to experimentally induced scurvy and produced swollen and bleeding gums, perifollicular hemorrhages, joint swelling and pain, conjunctival hemorrhages, and bilateral femoral neuropathy; results known for centuries.

The mentally handicapped have been subjects, too. A study designed to determine the infectiousness of hepatitis led researchers to artifically induce hepatitis in mentally handicapped children at an institution in which a mild form of the disease was accepted as endemic. Parents consented, but in some cases there was a clear suggestion that there would be no room for their children at the institution if they did not.[3] At a mental hospital in

Vietnam, an American psychiatrist tested aversive conditioning on Vietnamese schizophrenics. The mental patients were offered the choice of volunteering for a work program or submitting to unmodified electroconvulsive shock treatments. Those who accepted treatment and still refused to work were denied food for three days until they finally agreed to work.

Sick adults have been exploited. A study to determine portal circulation time and hepatic blood flow involved transcutaneous injection of the spleen and catheterization of the hepatic vein. Published reports made no mention of what estimation of the risks involved were given to the 43 subjects who participated, 14 of whom were well, the remainder already suffering from cirrhosis, acute hepatitis, and hemolytic anemia. In a study to test immunity to cancer, 22 hospitalized patients were injected with live cancer cells without being told that the cells were cancerous.

Persons motivated or compelled by their poverty have been used, well and sick. In a test of the effects of LSD, volunteers were paid $2 an hour to have their reactions to the drug observed, though no mention was made of the possible personality effects. Fifteen percent of the group had not even heard of the drug prior to the test. Although solid evidence was already available as to its effectiveness as a treatment of typhoid fever, chloramphenicol was withheld from 157 of 408 charity patients with typhoid fever. The death rate of the chloramphenicol treated group was 7.97 percent; of those receiving no chloramphenicol, 22.9 percent. This means that (approximately) 23 persons died to confirm this already well confirmed result.

And there have been cases in which the public has been used in an indiscriminate fashion. For example, a major group health plan conducted a pain tolerance test of 41,119 patients as part of their regular check-ups. Told only that it was a test of pressure tolerance, subjects placed their heels into a viselike machine until they could no longer stand the pain.

As morally troubling as these experiments appear, they pale in comparison with some of the outrages committed in the alleged interest of medical science during the second World War. No discussion of the abuses of human persons in medical experimentation can be complete in this century without mention of the abominations committed by Nazi medical experimentors against captive populations.[4] From small beginnings such as films depicting the alleged heroics of mercy killing and high school textbook problems requiring calculation of how many new housing units could be built for what it costs to care for the physically and mentally handicapped, the perverse Nazi ideology spread through the medical and scientific establishment. By 1936, only three years after Hitler's rise to power, extermination of the physically or socially unfit was so widely accepted that it was casually mentioned in an official German medical journal. By 1945, the full results of this disregard for the rights of human persons was revealed at the liberation of the concentration camps.

Gruesome and mutilating experiments with methods of sterilization were conducted on male and female prisoners without their knowledge or against their wills. The search for effective blood coagulants led Nazi experimenters to shoot Russian prisoners of war through the spleen to measure rates of bleeding. Human beings were dissected alive underwater to examine the effects of explosive decompression. To study treatment for exposure, humans were systematically frozen to death. The effects of an exclusive diet of unaltered sea water was tested on a group of Gypsies. Transplantation techniques were explored by removing healthy limbs from some humans and by attempting to reattach them to others. The use of sulfonamides against gangrene was tested by creating wounds and deliberately infecting them. In the alleged interest of science, a professor of anatomy at the University of Strassburg had 150 Jews murdered so that their skeletons could be preserved against the expected extinction of that entire group. And the list of like atrocities goes on.

One of the most disturbing aspects of this low point in human history is the fact that prior to the Nazi period, German society had largely the same religions, legal system, and social conventions that otherwise sustained western civilization. German medical schools were models imitated worldwide. German culture had produced a long series of outstanding scientists, artists, and philosophers. Yet in the space of twelve years, German physicians were banally reporting results of extermination techniques at medical meetings and were acting as executioners at the camps; German nurses were selecting troublesome patients at mental homes for extermination; and German university professors were accepting and encouraging scientific results gleaned from these barbarisms.

While we may never be able to provide anything like a complete account of this rapid and shocking moral decline, three conceptual aspects of the Nazi ideology were surely at the root of things: a racist genetic theory, a crassly instrumentalist view of the human person, and a political system hostile to democracy. The racist genetic theory held that not all persons were equal in worth. The crassly instrumentalist view was that the human person's worth was in his or her usefulness to the state. The political system's hostility to democracy consisted in the fact that political power was not broadly shared, individual moral rights were not respected legally, and the institutions and practices of society were closed to the free inspection, criticism, and participation of all its citizens. When these presumptions came into play in the context of medical experimentation, the morally unacceptable results we have seen above followed. Persons considered genetically inferior were thought to be useful only as things in the service of medicine and science; medicine and science themselves justified only by their service to the state. The moral demand that individual rights be acknowledged was swept aside as outdated and decadent. Abominations against persons and against whole groups were planned and conducted by a powerful few in institutions closed to public scrutiny. And, of course, there could be no such things as respect for human rights nor desire for the enhancement of practical personal autonomy in such a morally debased situation.

Among the lessons that we should take from this grisly Nazi period is that we renounce the ideals of autonomous persons in progressive societies at our own peril. The values of medical care and scientific advance will themselves be subverted if we weaken our commitment to the central and incalculable value of each human person and to the progressive societies in which persons are made to be autonomous and to thrive. These Nazi medical experiments provide an historically factual set of conditions under which scientific and medical progress is simply not worth having.

A second lesson we may take from both these American and Nazi experiments is that certain groups of persons are exceptionally vulnerable to abuse by medical science. These groups include children, prisoners, the mentally handicapped, the sick, and the poor. Each group is especially vulnerable to exploitation in the experimental context: children and the mentally handicapped because of their underdeveloped or impaired understandings; prisoners, the sick, and the mentally handicapped because of their likely institutionalization; prisoners and the poor because inducements of parole and money can impair the freedom of their wills; and all of them because they are in extraordinary relationships of dependence. This unusual state of dependence places a corresponding ethical burden upon the researcher who would use members of these groups as subjects. It will be useful to briefly review some of the additional ethical considerations relevant to the use of each group as research subjects.

Adults, as we have already seen, have a special bond of trust with children. For their part, children have a right as persons to freedom from conditions that impair the full development of their human capacities, especially the development of their practical personal autonomies. It would seem on the face of things that children ought never to be used as research subjects.[5] Yet because of the peculiarities of children's bodies and because children often react differently to drugs than adults do, there are many needed experiments for which adults are not fit substitutes. And because of the deeply felt pathos of childhood disease and death, the imperative for pediatric research is a strong one. We may begin to adjudicate this conflict of moral intuitions by distinguishing between research that might have some therapeutic benefit for the child in question and research which is purely for the sake of the advance of medical knowledge in general. In the former case of therapeutic research, the medical researcher may properly accept a proxy or substituted informed consent from the child's parents or guardians. The parents or guardians in such a case are morally bound to choose, not on the basis of their own self-interest, but as they conscientiously believe the child would choose were he or she able to. Of course, an older, understanding child should be in a position to give or withhold consent in addition to the parent's consent and should be made as complete a participant in such a decision as is factually possible. The role of the child in giving or refusing consent will thus vary with the child's age and maturity. Nontherapeutic research involving risk to children would have to pass stricter scrutiny. The justification of such research would require that the perceived benefits of the experiment be exceptionally great, the risk to the child exceptionally small, and the proxy consent of parent or guardian beyond reproach. Justification might be made easier if the child were a member of a highly susceptible population for the disease being researched, as this would draw the research closer to the therapeutic because of the medical benefit which may accrue directly to the child subject. Still, our special obligations as adults to protect children in this delicate stage of their development as persons ought to take precedence over most attempted justifications of risky nontherapeutic research with child subjects.

Prisoners are a captive population in an ambience of distorted values and in institutional settings notoriously difficult to monitor. Explicit promises of better treatment or extra privileges, the expectation of earlier parole, and the coercions built into their very circumstances can lead prisoners to accept risks in medical experimentation they would likely not accept outside the prison setting, and can lead jailors to force prisoners into experimentation entirely against their wills. Because of the potential for abuses here, the use of prisoner subjects must be extremely circumscribed.[6] It is probably too much to outright forbid prisoner experimentation completely, since practically free and informed consent is not wholly impossible even in prison and because some prisoners may be genuinely motivated to compensate society for their crimes. But the use of prisoners generally and the offer of inducements for prisoner volunteers must be subject to close public scrutiny and terminated at the least suggestion of the abuse of prisoner's rights as human persons.

The mentally handicapped are no less human persons for their impairments since, on our account, being a human person with equal rights requires only that one be a member of the species. Since they cannot themselves give informed consent, any involvement with experimentation will demand proxy consent. This proxy consent should be limited to therapeutic experimentation, though exception might be made again for research likely benefiting the mentally handicapped as a class, for example, researches into the causes, prevention, and treatment of mental handicaps. Here again proxies must choose not in terms of self-interest, but on the basis of what they conscientiously believe their charge would choose were he or she capable of it.

The sick are in a special relationship with medical professionals and their exploitation as research subjects would seriously violate their rights as patients, compromise the moral commitments of the medical professionals involved, and damage the social trust upon which the medical professional-patient relationship relies. Therefore, it is only prudent that if the sick do volunteer for nontherapeutic research (and this may be an ennobling activity, especially for the terminally ill), those who provide them with medical care should be clearly separated from those with whom they conduct research. This will minimize conflicts of interest and prevent abuse of the sick person's dependence on medical support. With respect to therapeutic experimentation, the sick, of course, have the right to accept

146

or refuse participation. It should be noted, however, that the hopelessness of the terminally ill's situation is a powerful inducement to volunteer for therapeutic research. A responsible researcher must take greater care to secure an understanding consent in the face of such a powerful inducement. One additional point is necessary here. While it is often scientifically preferable to conduct double-blind experiments, i.e. experiments in which some subjects are given inert placebos as a control while others are given active drugs and the knowledge of who received which is denied the researcher; while this sort of experiment is often scientifically preferable, it is never morally permissible to knowingly withhold a suspected therapeutic benefit from the sick without their explicit consent.[7] Thus, here as elsewhere the goals of medical progress must be subordinated to the rights and practical personal autonomy of the human person.

Finally, the poor are more likely to accept risks in a medical experiment that they otherwise would not accept but for the offer of money. So long as money plays the important role that it does in our society in determining an individual's life opportunities, and so long as large portions of our population are relatively indigent, the potential will exist for financial exploitation in the experimental context.[8] While it does seem appropriate to offer some financial compensation to experimental subjects in light of the time donated and the inconvenience involved, when the incentive to participate in medical research is primarily financial, moral issues are clearly raised. It surely is a form of coercion, however subtle and indirect, to be compelled by one's poverty to volunteer for a medical experiment. When this poverty is joined, as it so often is in our society, by racial discrimination, poor education, and lack of access to quality medical care, we are perilously close to exchanging the poverty stricken person's human dignity for a thing's price. For this reason, it is best if our financial compensations are never made so large as to become the primary inducement for participation in medical research.

C. Acceptable Human Research

As we have already made clear, the first and paramount condition for establishing the moral acceptability of using human persons for medical research is that these persons be genuine volunteers. This notion of voluntary participation can be extended to cover cases of proxy consent given on behalf of those who are incapable of giving or withholding consent themselves. These extensions must be made with great care and must themselves be bound by the moral limits of all proxy consent: The third party must choose in a way expressive of the best interests of the person chosen for. While it may seem initially implausible that the securing of medical results from a nontherapeutic experiment could ever be deemed to be in the best interest of some noncompetent subject, one might accept the claim that persons have a general interest in the groups to which they belong, including even society as a whole, but only when the risks involved in such nontherapeutic experiments are very small, the perceived benefits to the group involved very great, and there is no apparent self-interest operating on the part of the third party chooser. With this hedged exception for proxy consent, an exception which needs careful monitoring because of its obvious potential for abuse, the first and most important condition for the moral acceptability of research using human subjects is the genuine informed consent of the subjects involved. But there are other conditions as well, conditions which go beyond this minimal duty to insure that other important human values are preserved in the experimental context.[9]

A second condition is the earnest moral conscience of the experimentor, a conscience which exercises its own moral intuitions and wills those intuitions into action. This most general of moral conditions must be added to the requirement of informed consent since it is entirely possible that persons might volunteer for radically unconscionable experiments and might even do so with as complete an understanding and as free a will as is ever practically possible. But since the experimental context is not the subject's alone but a shared venture of the subject and the medical researcher together, the researcher's own moral conscience must delimit the range of experiments for which informed consent is even sought or accepted. There might, for instance, be persons who would knowingly volunteer to have a healthy limb removed and its reattachment attempted so as to research the role of the body's immune and rejection responses. There might be persons who would give informed consent to take even the most dangerous of new drugs or of new surgeries. There might even be persons who would knowingly and freely accept a terminal illness so that the conditions of their demise could be scientifically controlled and monitored. Who can say to what lengths persons might go to secure money for themselves or their families, attain fame and media recognition, or simply give their lives and deaths a new and exciting meaning? In light of these possibilities, subject informed consent is not enough. There must also be an earnest moral judgment on the part of the researcher, a judgment which rejects out of hand the sort of morally outrageous experiments conceived here. Again, this intuitive "knowing" is at the heart of all morality. Since no complete list or even approximation of a list of such morally outrageous experiments can be provided in advance of events, the continuously earnest moral conscience of the researcher must be relied upon to exercise itself in novel and unpredictable situations.

Thirdly, even when both of the above conditions prevail, an experiment involving humans may be morally unacceptable if it is scientifically inept. It is always wrong to risk the well-being of human persons, even when they volunteer, if the design of the experiment is so shoddy that nothing of medical significance can be learned. If human subjects are to be asked to assume risks in medical research, this request must be founded on the possibility of genuine advance in human knowledge relevant to medical care. Ill conceived or sloppily executed scientific experiments make genuine medical advance impossible and thereby jeopardize persons without justification. Thus, this condition requires that the morally responsible researcher be a professionally competent medical scientist as well.

148

Fourthly, the moral acceptability of human research requires that the degree of risk to human persons be proportionate to the significance of the medical knowledge sought. There can be no easy formula for determining appropriate risk; the earnest moral conscience of the researcher is required here again. But some cases can be obvious to all. Surely it would be wrong to risk the very life of a human subject to obtain trivial information or to reconfirm well secured information. Substantially risking a person's health in order to develop more effective hair dyes or to experimentally recreate small pox would be clear examples of risks not justified by anticipated results. Such examples and the many others like them that can be readily conjured up, underscore the need for the responsible researcher to refrain from initiating risks to other persons' health where too little can be learned to justify the degree of the risk. It is no response to this requirement to argue that the results of research are seldom wholly determinable at the outset of an experiment and that, for example, the development of new hair dyes might lead by whatever surprising route to a cure for cancer. While the history of medical science abounds with serendipitous discoveries, such good fortune cannot be made into an argument for risk taking for other persons when something of trivial human value is the immediate research objective. Morally acceptable medical experiments with human subjects must have reasonably clear goals and the risks entailed by the experiments must be proportionate to the direct significance of those goals for the improvement of medical care.

Fifth and finally, the earnest moral conscience of the researcher must be expressed not only in the rejection out of hand of morally outrageous experiments but it must also be expressed in a genuine indentification with the human subject as another person of equal and incalculably great value. This requires that the morally responsible researcher authentically believe that were he or she the experimental subject and the subject were the researcher, i.e., if roles were reversed, the researcher would accept as potential subject the risks the real subject is being asked to bear. As similar obligatory values, the researcher must be prepared to regard himself or herself and the subject similarly. This is an expression of the universalizing intent of morality and ethics. Furthermore, since such authentic beliefs, while absolutely central to the project of morality, are private and notoriously difficult to verify, the morally earnest medical researcher must make this private conviction public by demonstrating a willingness to allow public scrutiny of the experiment. Real public scrutiny is a practical check on privately imagined authenticity. A lesson from the history of medical experimentation is that many of the most morally objectionable experiments occurred in institutional settings removed from the public eye, in places like prisons, charity wards, and homes for the severely handicapped. The promotion of democratic habits in these institutions requires protection of the legal rights of their inhabitants and a structural openness to free inspection and participation by all citizens. The medical scientist need not actively seek publicity but neither should the public be denied access to the research in appropriate forums and on appropriate occasions. The morally responsible researcher must be willing imaginatively to reverse roles with the subject and practically to allow public scrutiny of his or her experiments. In this manner, the good will of the researcher is grounded both privately and publicly.

Morally acceptable research using human subjects must therefore involve the free and informed consent of subjects, a rejection of the morally outrageous, competent scientific procedures, proportionality in risk, and the private and public good will of the researcher. The moral burden of satisfying these conditions falls not only on the medical researcher but also on all health care professionals who participate in or who come to know about medical experiments involving human subjects. Because of the present ubiquity of medical experimentation and its likely continuance or increase in the future, the health care professional, even if not directly involved in research, will no doubt encounter numerous experiments involving human subjects. As the examples of U.S. experiments indicate, not all uses of human subjects can be expected to be ethically defensible even in our own nation. Moreover, as the examples of Nazi medical experimentation indicate, it is possible for whole social systems to become morally corrupt. This includes hospitals, universities, professions, and societies in general. If we are to protect and to enhance the practical personal autonomy of persons and build the progressive societies within which such autonomy thrives, all members of the medical professions must be vigilant against such individual and collective abuses.

A heavy responsibility therefore falls on the health care professional who encounters a medical experiment which he or she intuitively feels to be wrong. There are multiple conflicts of loyalties raised by such an event and many good reasons why such a professional bystander might be reluctant to act on this intuition. It is a natural, and in many respects laudable, human response to protect and defend one's professional colleagues. Surely no one would benefit from a situation in which team work and mutual professional support was damaged or destroyed because of the fear that one's colleagues were constantly and critically inspecting one's every professional move. Further, there are legally binding and ethically defensible levels of authority and decision-making competence in most health care and medical research settings. Physicians typically and rightfully have the final professional decision-making authority over the treatment of patients and over the testing of subjects as well.

Nevertheless, loyalty to one's professional colleagues can not justify disregard for the protection and enhancement of practical personal autonomy in the experimental context. This is as much true for health care professionals as it is for lawyers, police officers, elected officials, and for any group whose professional activities impinge directly on the real abilities of persons to defend and expand their practical autonomies. No health profession or scientific community is an elite freed from the general moral duties and value drives of all persons. To allow persons' rights to be violated or their potential for maximizing value attainments thwarted in a health care or research setting is not ethically different from allowing persons to be abused or dwarfed in one's own home, in the work place, or by government. The obligation to speak out on behalf of the exploited is not muted in any way by membership in a health care profession; indeed, if altered at all, the obligation is more strictly binding on the health care professional as he or she has freely taken on an additional commitment to the well-being of human beings.

While the chain of command model of authority and decision-making is legally and ethically defensible in the normal run of events, it cannot be made an excuse for ignoring one's personal moral obligations. There may be experts in medical treatment and in the design and execution of scientific research, but there are no moral experts. All persons must exercise their own moral intuitions of duty and of value, ethically clarify, organize, and criticize these intuitions, and will to do what they earnestly believe is right and good. The Allied trails of Nazi war criminals at Nuremberg after World War II established this ethical principle as an historical fact: No one is excused from their moral responsibilities by the command of a higher authority.[10] Similarly, no one is excused from the general moral duty to expose violations of human rights by the claim that someone of higher authority has commanded them not to. Again, there are no higher moral authorities; only our moral intuitions and our ethical reflections on them. When all the facts are available, the nurse, the pharmacist, the medical technician, and even the lay visitor on the hospital floor each has the same ability and responsibility to judge the moral acceptability of medical research with human subjects.

This is not to say that health care professionals must become detectives or that they should intrude upon experiments outside the range of their usual professional experience. Accepting the burden of one's moral responsibilities does not mean that one becomes offensive or indiscreet. Perhaps loyalty to one's colleagues entails that they be extended a presumption of ethical conduct until strong evidence suggests otherwise. Perhaps it also entails that one should first confront the investigator before pursuing a complaint publicly. It surely entails that no professional bystander take it upon himself or herself to subvert a colleague's research project without full knowledge of the project and without first consulting the relevant medical or scientific authorities. Having said this, however, the principle must be insisted upon: All health professionals, all persons, are obliged to speak out against assaults on human rights in the experimental setting. This is to say no more than that the health professional must be responsible, must be willing and able to respond to the moral challenges of his or her role.

The general public has responsibilities here as well. The moral disintegration of Nazi society was not initiated nor primarily carried by medical scientists, but by the public of that society as a whole. The corruption of its medical institutions was just one expression of the moral decay of all of the major institutions in German society. This historical fact underscores the need for continued and vigorous commitment to our moral ideals and especially to the building of progressive societies whose democratic habits of power sharing, protection of legal rights, and free citizen participation help to make the wholesale institutional abuse of persons less likely. The achievement of such progressive societies is primarily, but not exclusively, a political task as we have already seen. A society becomes stronger and less susceptible to such systematic abuses when democratic habits are built throughout all the various institutions, communities, and associations that make up a society. Protection and enhancement of the cultural achievements already embedded in our hospitals, universities, and health care professions require continued commitment to the maximization of practical personal autonomy through the building of democratic habits throughout these institutions and practices.

One final social dimension of medical research deserves mention. Although voluntary participation in needed and morally responsible medical experimentation goes well beyond any conceivable sense of duty, it does help to secure some vitally important human values. Such research expands the power of medicine and helps to increase human pleasure, happiness, and practical personal autonomy, or at least it helps to decrease their opposites. By free and knowing acceptance of risk, volunteers for human research offer part of themselves to secure these values for persons whom they have never and likely will never come to meet and know. Such willingness to sacrifice for unknown others on the part of a number of persons sufficiently large to sustain continued medical progress is a precious moral resource for any society. This moral resource should not be squandered through tolerance of abuses in the experimental context. On the contrary, if the conditions for the moral acceptability of medical research are made to prevail routinely in experimental contexts, then we should promote in our moral education of the young and of one another as adults, the feelings and habits that give rise to such self-sacrifice. The social production of large numbers of persons who earnestly and spontaneously go beyond the dictates of duty in this regard is the condition on which continued improvement of medical care depends and a mark of a whole society's moral excellence.

Chapter 12.

The New Genetics

A. The Prospect of Disease Omniscience

Our consideration of the contemporary hospital focused on present social dimensions of medicine and the discussion of medical research marked our social debts to the past. The last social dimension of medical care we shall consider points to the medicine of the future and the genetic interventions which future medicine will likely make possible. Though the evolution of the human body has had a long history, self-conscious human participation in that evolution is a novel part of today's medicine and one which will likely dominate ethical debate in the next century. We stand now on the edge of a medical revolution through which the skillful practitioner can become virtually all knowing with respect to genetically based and genetically related diseases. Through new genetic knowledge and power, physicians of the future may become nearly disease omniscient. This disease omniscient practitioner of the future will be able to readily identify those who surely will suffer from a genetically based disease; those who will not themselves suffer from such a disease but who are likely to bear children who will; and those who are highly susceptible to a genetically related disease. Though there are other environmental factors which come into play in diseases which are not directly caused by our genes but only significantly related to them, this susceptibility to genetic disease can and will be determined with a high degree of probability on the basis of the presence of certain biomarkers in the body, biomarkers which are statistically correlated with the later onset of the genetically related disease in question.

The attainment of such a state of virtual omniscience with respect to genetic disease is not a wildly speculative possibility, but a probability based upon a reasonable extrapolation from what is already a matter of fact.[1] At present, we can identify a number of genetic defects before birth through amniocentesis, a technique which taps the amniotic fluid surrounding the fetus *in utero*. Down's syndrome, for example, can be readily identified by amniocentesis. Other genetic problems can also be identified at or soon after birth. Phenylketonuria (PKU), for example, can be identified by a simple analysis of an infant's urine sample; as can other genetically based metabolic disorders such as galactosemia, homocystinuria, tyrosinemia, and histideinemia. The list of genetic diseases which can be identified through techniques such as fetal amniocentesis and neonatal urine and blood samplings grows annually and may reasonably be expected to continue indefinitely. At the same time, work continues on techniques for the early identification of subjects of genetic diseases having a late adult expression, such as Huntington's chorea. There are now reliable tests to identify carriers (heterozygotes) of some genetic diseases who, because of the genetic structure of the diseases involved (autosomal recessive, for example), will not themselves express the disease in their own bodies, but whose offspring are at high risk to suffer from it. Tay-Sachs disease and sickle cell anemia are two examples of genetic diseases whose mechanism for transfer to the next generation is relatively clear and predictable already. Finally, evidence is mounting that the presence of certain biomarkers in the body, for example, some kinds of histocompatibility (HLA) antigens, blood cholesterol, and other lipids, are highly predictive of the later development of cancers, heart diseases, and other illnesses. These biomarkers appear to have a significant hereditary component.[2] Given these realities, and especially given the comparative youth of this field of medical investigation, can it be unreasonable to expect that, with the exception of accident, malnutrition, ambient toxicity, unusual life styles, and other clearly environmental variables, the future holds the promises and perils of near disease omniscience at birth or even at conception itself? If this expectation is correct, future parents will have a staggering range of genetic probabilities available with respect to their future offspring and they will have available after conception or birth a blueprint of their child's future disease history, other environmental factors being equal.

What will be the moral implications of such knowledge? Will it always be a good thing to know one's future diseases? What if one knows of the inevitability of some disease for which there is no effective treatment; the personal losses are graphic here, but the gains obscure. Whose knowledge will this disease omniscience be? If it is the parents', how will this influence the parent-child relationship? When and how will the child be told, and what will be the effects of knowing? What will be the effects of the availability of such knowledge on insurance carriers, employers, friends, and mates? Can this knowledge be keep confidential in this day of third party payers and computer storage of information? If it cannot be kept confidential, will individuals already suffering from the knowledge of their future diseases be made victims of social stigmatization as well? Will we be calculating the future costs of certain racial or ethnic groups at high risk for expensive to treat diseases? Will there be single issue interest groups of those who know they may be future victims of certain diseases? Will there be legally compelled screening to force each of us to provide this bodily information, or will we be free to keep others and ourselves in ignorance about our bodies' disease futures? Will there be a national registry of disease histories to be? If so, would potential spouses have a right of access to knowledge of their lover's future diseases? If parents have a right to genetic ignorance, can their genetically impaired offspring recover legal damages against their parents for wrongful life? Will society refuse to allow some genetically high risk couples to marry at all, or mandate sterilization of carriers of genetic disease before marriage? Will those susceptible to specific future diseases be forced by law, insurance carriers, or the tyranny of public opinion to adopt certain life-styles which lower the environmental support for the triggering of their genetically related

154

disease mechanisms? When we are thus omniscient, how will we come to think of ourselves and others; specifically, will our hard won presumption of human equality yield to new class structures and divisions among persons based on persons' future diseases and their costs?

These and similar questions can be generated indefinitely since the prospect of such new genetic knowledge works a dramatic change in our bodily self-understanding and on our relationships with one another. While it cannot be part of this reflection to address all these issues, a useful start can be made by focusing attention directly on a human relationship of historical significance which will be influenced early and strongly by this approaching social reality: the doctor-patient relationship. The drama of the questions above can be scaled down to more manageable proportion by locating them specifically against this important relationship between a physician and patient. For example, can a physician obtain a morally valid informed consent from a patient for a disease omniscience test? Can any patient ever understand the full implications of such knowledge and completely and freely will to have it? Will the disease omniscient physician of the future be morally bound to tell the patient everything, even in cases where the prognosis indicates a horrible and untreatable disease? Can the release of such information possibly fall within the ambit of the traditional medical ethics prescription of **primum, non nocere,** or will doctors of the future be directly harming patients with this information, even filling mental institutions or driving up the suicide rate with their scientific prophesies? Can such information be kept within the traditional bounds of confidentiality in the doctor-patient relationship, or will the pressures that will likely come from government officials, scientific researchers, and insurance actuaries breach these traditional bounds? Will the disease omniscient physician have the counseling skills to match these new powers? Even if the physician has such competence, what standards will be used to help patients reach crucial decisions about parenting, about life-style, about preventive measures? Most importantly, can such an all knowing physician retain the traditional fiduciary relationship by continuing to act for the best interests of that individual patient? Indeed, who will be the patient of this future physician — an individual, future generations, or society as a whole? And if such ambiguity is introduced into the doctor-patient relationship, can we even hope to maximize practical personal autonomy through the attainment of therapeutic relationships of mutual participation?

If we are to maintain the moral achievements already embodied in the doctor-patient relationship and medical care generally in the face of this new knowledge, vigorous democratic social habits will have to be developed to control the collection, possession, and use of disease omniscience.[3] This new genetic knowledge will give individual doctors and medicine collectively unheralded power. If we are to contain this power within reasonable limits and so protect the vulnerability of patients and the public, there must be political sharing of this power, legal protection of persons against it, and the widest possible citizen participation in the institutions and practices relevant to this information's collection, possession, and use. As in all cases of value maximization, this last element of citizen participation will be a highly creative one, but one necessary element of such participation is already clear. If such progressive control over new genetic knowledge and power is to be possible, the public must be educated in genetics and to the potential of our impending knowledge and power to a degree unthinkable even in our recent past. Doctors in their professional organizations and at the local level must take the lead in advocating measures to assure the responsible use of disease omniscience. Doctors must be teachers and leaders in this collective educational effort.

Even as they take part in a wider democratic social effort, doctors must become increasingly sensitive to the moral and legal rights of their individual patients in genetics related medical contexts. Indeed, it would also seem appropriate that doctors become leaders in the articulation of claims for the new moral and legal rights which these new facts make both possible and necessary in light of our ideals of autonomous persons in progressive societies. The new power which doctors will have can make them more effective agents for their individual patients' value interests, more effective in producing pleasure, happiness, and practical personal autonomy through the genetic wellness they can bring. On the other hand, this new power can make doctors parties to the exploitation and alienation of patients for the sake of the alleged common good of our gene pool as a whole. Only by a self-conscious redoubling of commitment to individual patients can doctors insure the former and avoid the latter. Doctors must reaffirm their historical fiduciary relationship with their individual patients in the face of disease omniscience and avoid becoming genetic risk-benefit calculators.

From a political perspective, disease omniscience offers us the power to share directly and self-reflectively in our own biological evolution. The genetic dispositions we have inherited individually and collectively represent, as we have seen, a physical sedimentation of centuries of human and prehuman experience. In light of the vast time period through which these vehicles of information have come to us, a conservative stance toward tampering seems appropriate. This means that we must resist through our democratic political institutions any and all attempts to create a positive eugenics programs, that is, attempts to chart a course for the artificial improvement of our species inheritance. Of course, in individual cases of genetic defect, there is a strong moral imperative to intervene for the sake of prevention, cure, or management. Individual human lives are short and filled with the pathos of events, events often strongly shaped by genetic dispositions. The demand to aid these human beings by directly removing or palliating genetic disease and by preventing more disease through individual counseling; this demand is as compelling as any in medicine. Nevertheless, as members of a species in a delicately balanced ecological niche (itself under unprecedented pressures), the path of political wisdom seems to lie in deference to the long successes of nature. Thus, as we approach disease omniscience, the political burden of proof ought always to be borne by those who advocate positive interventions to produce genetically ideal persons or an ideal gene pool. Not only are such notions vague in themselves, since who can say what the ideal human person or gene pool should be like, but they also strike a note of elitism and authoritarianism, themes incompatible with the pluralism and equality implied by our ideals of autonomous persons in progressive societies. In this respect, the doctors' **primum** principle should govern our political and social policies regarding genetics as well: first, we should do no harm. Only in this manner can we introduce human moral judgment into the otherwise inexorable logic of technology uncontrolled; a logic which may drive us to do genetically everything that can be done, whether or not it should be done.

A more detailed exploration of the factual possibilities at hand and the impact they will likely have on the ideals, values, and duties we have espoused here will provide one final opportunity to assert the central thesis of this reflection: Reality is a subtle interplay of changing facts and evolving ideals. Morality and ethics are our tools to help shape reality ever more in line with our ideals as we understand and feel them. But here as elsewhere, serious attention to the changing world of fact and its implications for our ideals is a necessary step before any reasonable course of action animated by our ideals is possible.

B. The Perils of Disease Omniscience

As we approach genetic disease omniscience, pressures will be brought to bear on the ideals, values, and duties that compose the moral dimensions of the doctor-patient relationship. The imperative to achieve such knowledge in any given case, the desire to have it in all cases, and the multiple practical possibilities implicit in disease omniscience will challenge respect for patients' rights, the primacy of the **primum** principle, and the fiduciary demand that doctor's act to serve the best interests of their patients. Thus, these new facts in genetics contain the peril of eroding practical personal autonomy in medical contexts.

Respect for persons' rights as has been characterized here will be difficult to maintain should persons become thought of as merely vehicles for the conveyance of genetic information; a deterioration already anticipated by the notion of an individual person as a "carrier" of genetic defects. A wholesale move in this direction means the reduction of a person to a thing, reduction of a being of incalculably great value to a transmission instrument with a value relative to the information carried. There is also the more specific danger of relativizing the value of persons on the basis of the costs of the diseases they will express or convey to others. One can easily foresee the possibility that an early detection of a likely cancer victim might cause that future victim additional present suffering if he or she comes to be thought of in terms of the price of the treatments eventually required. When price becomes a dominant concern, mandatory screening for genetic disease and mandatory registering of all genetic dispositions

157

will appear to be reasonable cost control mechanisms. Truth and confidentiality in the relationship with the individual persons screened and registered may even appear to be a luxury which society can ill afford, especially since the mere collection and storage of such information may not itself constitute a doctor-patient relationship in the strict legal sense. Finally, there is the obvious danger of moving, however slowly and subtly, from the emotive categories of sympathy to those of resentment when thinking of victims of genetically related disease: **They** cost **us.** The next step in decline could be the stigmatization of the biological victim as a social problem and the consequent branding of those persons as somehow less worthy than those of greater genetic fortune. Disease omniscience portends a future which may hold the transvaluation of persons to things, to things of relative value, and to things whose relative value is not equal to the higher value of others.

The **primum** principle itself may be challenged by the advent of disease omniscience. The prospects of a dramatic reduction or elimination of genetically based and genetically related diseases may become so attractive and the public clamor for them so irresistible, that direct harms will be done to patients to bring about this great good. We may in the future harm persons by compromising their practical personal autonomy through the demand, perhaps with the force of law, that they yield up their genetic disease futures to public collection and inspection whether they want to or not. This coercion would itself be a direct moral harm and it may be perpetrated by or with the assistance of physicians or other health care professionals. The individual patient may also be harmed by being given genetic information whose only significant medical upshot is increased personal anxiety and negative fixation on future bodily ills. In this sense, early prediction of genetic disease, especially when no treatment is available, may itself be a cause of sickness. Early knowledge of one's future diseases may even lead to the harms of mental breakdown and suicide. Harm may also be done if such information about a patient's disease future becomes publicly available so that it affects the patients ability to secure employment, carry insurance, or lead a normal life generally. The release of such information may harm patients even if it is restricted to intimate circle of family and relatives; it can impair such important relationships by the introduction of adverse elements of pity, guilt, or shame. Finally, grave harms can be envisioned by considering the practical imperatives of disease omniscience. Such knowledge holds out the possibility of genetic selection, i.e., the systematic preference for some types of genetic expressions in human bodies over others. In its wholesale positive expression, genetic selection means a eugenics program in which we seek to create the perfect person or the perfect gene pool. Such an attempt portends serious harms to those judged less perfect themselves or likely to bear less perfect children. A negative expression of such a drive to artifically improve our genetic information could take the form of forced sterilization of carriers of genetic diseases, directly impairing these persons' practical personal autonomy. More likely, a negative genetic selection program, one designed to eliminate defects rather than produce perfection, will take the form of increased use of therapeutic abortion, the destroying of fetuses judged not fit by some genetic standard. This practice, based on amniocentesis, is already widely used to destroy fetuses known to have Down's syndrome. Since we have already attentuated the concept of therapy here by allowing it to include the destruction of the subject of the disease, there is every likelihood that pressures will arise to use therapeutic abortion to eliminate subjects of a wide range of genetically based and genetically related diseases. There might even develop social pressures on parents to accept it as their genetic responsibility to abort all fetuses conceived to be less than perfect by reference to some social standard. Who can gauge the dimensions of the harms implied here? The results of such an abortion policy might even be good genetically, but this good will be had at the cost of doing great harm. These harms will include the taking of the very lives of those judged to be insufficiently perfect, the diminution of parents' practical autonomy, and, no doubt, considerable public confusion, hypocrisy, and self-deception caused by the embrace of the vague and perhaps empty notion of genetic perfection.

If such a deteriorated moral situation were to come to pass, the doctor-patient relationship will have changed its character in a dramatic way: the fiduciary nature of the relationship will have been lost. The doctor will have become an agent of the government, of insurance carriers, or of some eugenics program itself in the service of an indefinite future gene pool. The centrality of the individual patient at hand will have been abandoned as concrete personal relationships of mutual participation are replaced by active-passive relationships of genetic manipulation. The medical geneticist may even come to regard his or her patient as the whole of society, future generations, or the gene pool itself. If the patient is conceived to be these collective entities, confidential protections for the individual patient will likely give way to the alleged common good and concern for the individual patient's best interest will yield to the interests of the whole of society and its future. The standards used in patient genetic counselling may then shift from those of the patient to those of the society at large, a shift from the person centered to the group centered.

This is a most unpleasant scenario of what the future may hold in store for us. It is not described here to express hostility to science or cynicism about medicine. On the contrary, acknowledgement of the dangers which the future may hold is a simple act of a common sense which admits that any great boon to humanity has an equally great potential for abuse. The willingness to anticipate such abuse so as to control them is a mark of human intelligence, an intelligence coextensive with the mind of science and the heart of medicine.

Against these dire possibilities must also be placed the assertion that any knowledge which provides us with the ability to prevent and minimize some significant sources of human sufferings is a positive value. It is a genuinely good thing to eliminate genetic defects, since these defects severely debilitate persons and their offspring and thus subvert the development of practical personal autonomy. And they cause great suffering and pain. It is a good thing to help people minimize the likelihood of having genetically defective offspring by giving them information that might lead them to interventions to permit conception and gestation without defect, adoption, or the choice not to have children at all. It is a good thing to warn people of genetically related susceptibilities to disease so that they can take reasonable steps to minimize this likelihood or to rationally alter their life-styles in preparation for it. Finally, it is a good thing, in fact a responsibility, to be concerned for the well-being of entities larger than the person; families, communities, society both present and future. These entities contain in their social habits the accomplishments of persons in the past and set the horizon against which persons of the future will develop their own feelings, habits, and abilities to be practically autonomous. Furthermore, without the selfless concern of physicians, scientists, and citizens alike for these organic social entities in the past, our health, collectively and as individual persons, would be much worse than the standards we have come to enjoy today. There is indeed a weighty value imperative here to increase what we know, to grow in power, and to use that knowledge and power for maximizing the pleasure, happiness, and practical personal autonomy of future generations of human persons. If we are to do justice to this value imperative, then the drive to attain disease omniscience must be pursued and new ways of using this power for the relief and improvement of humanity must be developed continuously. Nevertheless, we cannot seek to maximize these human values until our duties to the value of values have been acknowledged and discharged. These duties are structured into the equal rights we have admitted for all persons and into the doctor-patient relationship specifically. If we are to have these values and discharge these duties together, we must evolve standards for the collection, possession, and use of this genetic knowledge. These standards must be such that they preserve the best of our established values and duties while they accommodate new knowledge and new powers; in short, standards that preserve and refine our ideals in the light of new facts.

Before describing some specific elements which any acceptable set of standards must embody if they are to accommodate our ideals with fact and vice versa, the most obvious general conditions must be stated clearly at the outset. They are two. The first condition is that the doctrine of informed consent as the central expression of practical personal autonomy in the medical context must be brought into the disease omniscient doctor-patient relationship. However the factual specifics of that relationship may change in light of new knowledge and power, this crucial protection of the patient as the incalculably worthy source of value creative activity must be a fundamental of all therapeutic relationships. The many goods available personally and socially through disease omniscience will not be worth having if this key element is lost or overshadowed in the doctor-patient relationship of the future.

Secondly, physicians must continue to attempt to create relationships of mutual participation with their genetics patients, relationships which will assure a trustful, confidential, and empathetic context for the care of genetic disease. There is a potential for arrogance contained in increased knowledge, increased power, and even in the relationship of the healthy to the sick in general. This potential for arrogance must be tempered by a keen awareness of the chance character of genetically based and genetically related wellness and sickness. The physician's personal concern for the patient must arise out of a profound awareness that no one of us has deserved or merited in any fashion the genetic inheritance we have received. We each find ourselves in families and with bodies that we did not ask for nor earn. Furthermore, we each carry from three to five severely mutant genes which we may well pass on to our own descendents.[4] Sympathy for those whose lot appears to be less than ours is nurtured by deepening an appreciation for the common lot of all human persons and for the mystery of the distribution of life's opportunities and woes. There is no room for arrogance in a geneticist who sees a common humanity in his or her patient and who habitually feels and understands that the gulf which separates their lives' prospects is one which is beyond all human comprehension and blame. The fiduciary responsibility of the physician to act for the best interests of patients is finally grounded in natural piety in the face of an incalculably valuable person. This natural piety must permeate our use of new genetic knowledge and new genetic powers.

With these moral prerequisites, we can now describe what elements any guidelines for the moral control of disease omniscience must have if they are to be useful in securing the promise of this new power and in protecting us from its peril, that is, if they are to be useful in maximizing practical personal autonomy.

C. Promise Without Peril

We can organize this discussion of the necessary moral elements of guidelines for the control of future disease omniscience by reference to the moral categories which will likely undergo the most social pressure to change in unacceptable ways. First, we will describe certain necessary moral elements for guidelines that can preserve patients' rights as human persons. Second, we will describe those elements that can preserve and enhance medicine's commitment to the **primum**, to first doing no harm. Finally, we will describe the necessary moral elements of guidelines that can preserve and enhance the fiduciary character of the physician's relationship with his or her individual patients.

If we are to preserve patients' rights as human persons in genetics contexts, we must above all insist on the equal and incalculably great value of each human person. The attempt to reduce a patient to the costs we know their treatment will mean to society is a direct violation of the absolute value and consequent dignity which we have attributed to all persons. However we collectively determine the subsequent distribution of inevitably scarce medical resources, persons ought not to become relative values in genetic risk-benefit calculations for reasons that we have already reviewed. Disease omniscience may well bring with it a heightened sense of the overwhelming price of health care interventions generally, but we must resist the temptation to develop a disaster or triage mentality in our day to day doctor-patient encounters. Such a triage mentally would mean that some of the worst, most expensive cases of genetic defect should get no treatment at all so that more of the available funds can be diverted to the promising cases. Triage has its role in the face of genuine disaster, such as those typical of military medicine. But when applied to ordinary medical care, a triage mentality can only mean the moral disaster of ranking the relative values of persons.[5] We must not count persons' values by reference to the facts of the expenses of their diseases but must continue to insist on the right of each person to be regarded and treated as an incalculably worthy sources of value creative activity.

Secondly on the score of preserving patients' rights, because one of the important bases upon which this lofty ideal appraisal of the human person depends is the potential of persons for practical autonomous decision-making, persons must not be coerced. In spite of the attractiveness of these ideas, we must resist all and any attempts to politically impose mandatory genetic screening, genetic counseling, registration of genetic information, sterilization, therapeutic abortion, and adjustment in life-style due to high susceptibility to genetically related disease.[6] Exceptions to this principle may have to be made when dealing with groups genuinely incapable of practical autonomous decision-making (mandatory PKU testing of infants seems to be a reasonable exception, for example). But since there is a decided tendency in human psychology to expand the category of those deemed incapable of practical autonomy to include all those who disagree with one's own reasoning, exceptions to this rule should be well defined and clearly justified.

Finally, patients are incapable of practical personal autonomy and thus are robbed of a key element of their rights as persons when they are denied access to important truths about themselves. While there is no clear imperative that a physician tell a patient everything known or suspected about his or her condition, when a patient requests it, that patient must be given the truth of his or her genetic dispositions. This may be an increasingly difficult and painful prescription as we approach disease omniscience, but nothing subverts a person's practical autonomy more thoroughly or destroys the context of truth in the doctor-patient relationship more rapidly than lying or dissembling.[7] Even when the next of kin alone is provided the truth, the act of deceiving a patient takes its toll since that next of kin too will someday have to rely on a physician's word; and the experience of a prior conspiracy of deceit will surely impair the character of that doctor-patient relationship. We must insist that maximization of practical personal autonomy requires recognition of the right of patients to have access on demand to all information acquired about their individual disease futures.

Preservation and enhancement of the traditional medical **primum** will require considerable attention as the prospect of genetic disease omniscience brings a new meaning to the colloquial chestnut that "ignorance is bliss." Bliss it may never really be, but ignorance of the future, especially of future disease, can be an important psychic refuge in the present. In many ways, the present just is what it is because of the imponderability of the future. When the future becomes determined and closed to imaginative adjustments, one's sense of freedom and hope can easily give way to resignation and despair. Even though it may often be foolish to exercise such a right, we will have to admit that persons have a right not to be harmed in the present by being forced to receive information about their future sicknesses. Only by the acknowledgement of such a right can we prevent the logic of disease omniscience from expanding future harms into present harms as well. This does not mean that it will not be generally good to know of future disease likelihoods so as to allow for preventive measures in the present, nor does it entail that we ought not to take educational steps to put persons in a better emotional position to handle such information. What it does entail is that if some persons, for whatever reasons, elect not to know what disease they will likely suffer from, then those persons have the right not to know. To force such knowledge on persons would be to inflict direct and grave personal harms and would thus violate the principle of first doing no harm.

This element has a further practical implication. As disease omniscience draws near, there will likely be great pressure to screen for all genetically based and genetically related diseases to provide a data base for research. As reasonable a desire as this is, it must be moderated by the interests of the persons involved and by the **primum.** There may be good scientific reasons but there is no clear medical justification for screening for diseases for which there is no available treatment and no preventive measures open to the subject of those diseases. While there are some diseases whose genetic transfer is so clear that alteration of one's reproductive intentions may itself be considered prevention (Huntington's chorea, for example), generally we ought not to test for the presence of untreatable diseases nor use multiphasic tests which include tests for untreatable diseases. If there genuinely is nothing a soon to be affected individual can do to prevent or manage a future disease, then there is no good reason to burden that person with the knowledge of the inevitability of the disease unless that person freely and knowingly seeks such knowledge. Perhaps there will be a day when there is no such inevitability, a day when all genetically based and genetically related diseases will be open to some meaningful therapy or prevention. Short of that day however, the unrequested giving of all knowing forecasts without the giving of any reasonable medical hope is a harm to patients without justification.

A second **primum** related element has to do with harms that may be caused by others. Not only can the knowledge of one's future diseases be a direct harm to the individual person, it can also be an indirect but real harm when others have access to this knowledge. Because we know that such knowledge can negatively and wrongfully affect a person's employment, ability to obtain insurance, family life, and relationships with other persons, the affected person must maintain complete control over who has access to information about his or her future disease. The physician must hold information about a patient's future in strictest confidence to avoid being a party to these harms. Above all, such knowledge must be kept out of computer storage where its confidentiality cannot be assured. If portions of this information must be so stored (as a public health record, for example), it ought to be purged of individual names and identities. This policy will maintain the trust in individual doctor-patient relationships, and will also guard against the social deterioration of the relationship in general. It will take few instances of the public display of an individual's private disease dispositions to keep the general public away from all voluntary genetic screening and counseling programs. Harms then would have extended from the persons whose futures are wrongfully opened to the public, to society as a whole, which, because of these revelations, may deny itself the real benefits available through voluntary use of new genetic knowledge and power.

The final element in guidelines needed to protect and expand the medical **primum** is a total ban on mandatory eugenics programs. Persons must not be harmed by being coerced into altering their reproductive activities because of some socially defined goal of an improved or perfect generation of persons in the future. Forced sterilization or limitation of any sort on a competent adult's ability to have children is too clearly a frustration of that person's practical autonomy and too clearly a source of personal suffering to permit on our ethical principles. In light of the very vagueness inherent in the idea of factual bodily perfection and in light of the number of genetic defects each person carries recessively, pursuit of genetic perfection will likely bring other personal and social harms in its wake, harms which can be avoided entirely if we renounce the whole notion of the genetically perfect.[8]

Without raising directly the difficult moral issue of abortion, another concern here is the prospect that therapeutic abortion will become the major practical implication of disease omniscience. One's sympathy with the pathos of an abortion decision in the face of a severe genetic defect in the fetus wanes as one moves away from the prevention of the tragic and toward creation of the perfect. Already there are reports of abortions performed because the fetus had the misfortune of being the wrong sex for the parents' family plans.[9] As our information from amniocentesis approaches disease omniscience, parents to be may increasingly demand a "genetically perfect" child. Since this category of the genetically perfect is virtually empty, abortions performed on this basis will be performed without a meaningful criterion and will more than likely reflect the arbitrariness of parents' whims and social fashions. Even if such decision-making never reaches the absurdities of preferred height, eye color, and shape of the nose, we will surely confront therapeutic abortion decisions made on the basis of life expectancy and morbidity. Will future parents abort a child who will likely develop cancer in his or her teens, or in the twenties, thirties, or forties? The prospect of such dilemmas generated beneath the chimerical goal of genetic perfection ought to lead us to insist that we not use therapeutic abortion as a means of seeking the genetically perfect child. The harm to the "less than perfect" fetus is too graphic and the social implications too portentious to permit such a eugenics policy. The drive for factual perfection in this matter is a short step away from a total devaluing of the imperfect. Such a drive ought to be moderated considerably by the frank admission that no one of us is more than imperfect genetically. Perfection can be a part of our ideals but it can never display itself fully in fact. The notion of factual genetic perfection is therefore bound to be a will-o-the-wisp and a potent source of great harms.

The fiduciary character of the doctor-patient relationship must also be defended and strengthened by guidelines to control our new genetic knowledge and power. This means that the medical geneticist must be the agent for his or her patient directly and not for any larger entities. It is a matter of fact that most of the vast improvement in health standards and longevity in this century has been due not to individual medical interventions, but to improvements in nutrition, sanitation, and the public's awareness of health hazards.[10] In many respects, medical genetics shares more in common with such public health and preventive measures than it does with conventional individual relationships. This is so because our genetic inheritance may be so readily conceived as a public domain, even as the notion "gene pool" suggests. Because of this, there will likely be pressures on the genetically disease omniscient physician to become the agent of the public, the government, or the gene pool itself. This pressure must be resisted if doctor-patient relationships of mutual participation are to be maximized, and especially if the central fiduciary responsibility of the medical professional to protect the practical personal autonomy of patients is to be sustained and developed. Physicians must not become agents of the state, the future gene pool, or any third party in addition to the individual patient served. Physicians may indeed have public responsibilities as physicians to help shape intelligent genetics policies at the political level. We may be approaching a day of third party payments for all health services or even a national health service in which many physicians are paid directly by the state. Nevertheless, the primary moral relationship in medicine has been and ought to remain that between one human person as doctor and one human person as patient. Only in this way can patients be assured that their own best interest is foremost in their physician's decision-making.

A second element pertinent to the fiduciary responsibility of the physician has to do with his or her new role as a genetic counselor. Accurate and sensitive transmission of the fruits of disease omniscience to patients will require considerable counseling skills on the part of physicians. Surely it is part of the role of the physician as genetic counselor to help make patients aware of the possibilities at hand, including various dimensions of persons' social responsibilities and obligations to future generations. Still, the final reproductive decisions of a patient as a practically autonomous person ought to be made on the basis of his or her own values. It is not enough for the physician to simply tell this to the patient. Patients are notoriously deferential to doctors' advice and can easily be led to make decisions thought pleasing to the doctors on whom they so much depend. In light of this, genetic counselling should be as nondirective and as free of the physician's own biases as is humanly possible. A physician faced with a patient whose values on these matters are morally repugnant may rightfully invite that patient to seek another professional, but in general the physician should assume the role of supplier of information and options and not that of decision-maker. The best interests of a competent adult person are always served by enlarging that person's practical personal autonomy through the exercise of free and reasonable choice.

Finally, the fiduciary character of the doctor-patient relationship can be preserved and enhanced if doctors take the lead in defending those of their patients who suffer from genetic disease. As disease omniscience is approximated, the human inclination to ostracize and abuse the different will be given new energy. It has taken human persons and societies centuries to reach today's relative tolerance of persons who appear different from the majority. Even within this modest cultural achievement, there has arisen the recent Nazi genetic theory of value; there is the daily fact of subtle and not so subtle racism and sexism; and there is still the common morbid fascination and hostility at the birth of infants with genetically based malformations. It would be naive to think that nearly complete knowledge of our future genetic diseases could not create new categories of genetic pariahs. But this unhappy result is not inevitable. Physicians are in a position to help contain the stereotyping of individuals by the provision of accurate information about our genetic inheritance and by reminding us all of our own genetic vulnerabilities. Above all, physicians must be in the forefront of attempts to prevent the stigmatization of patients who are already victims of genetic diseases. As professionals close to their patients' sufferings, physicians must take the lead in reducing such sufferings and ought never to allow their work to contribute to the blaming of the victim. Such concern for the genetically sick is a natural extension of the doctor's responsibility to seek to serve the best interests of his or her patients.

Incorporation of these elements into guidelines to control the acquisition and use of new genetic knowledge will not of itself guarantee that this knowledge is collected, possessed, and used responsibly. Here as everywhere, one must depend on the earnest moral conscience of the persons most directly involved. But as we have seen, that earnest moral conscience develops and operates from a background horizon of personal and social feelings and habits, feelings and habits which can themselves be built and rebuilt in light of ideals and the values and duties we derive from them. The future of these issues is in the hands of those who will choose tomorrow, but the building of the moral feelings and habits out of which those choices will issue is in our hands today. If we build the right feelings and habits so that we will intuitively feel and think in accord with our ideals of autonomous persons in progressive societies, then those ideals will not be the pious but empty dreams some have taken them to be. Instead, they will be the ideal vision on the basis of which the fact world of tomorrow's genetics is remade and a new more humanly ideal reality created, a reality which serves to maximize human pleasure, happiness, and the attainment of practical personal autonomy.

Epilogue: Ideal, Fact, and Medicine

It is appropriate that we take a retrospective look at what has been claimed in this work. Philosophical reflection is able, by its very nature, to isolate aspects from the unity of lived experience. The major aspects of reality are the world of our human ideals and the world of fact, and there are multiple and subtle relationships between them. Among the ideals factually available to us in this culture at this time are the ideals of autonomous persons in progressive societies. We have embraced those ideals here on the basis of what are at root four reasons.

The first two reasons are primarily ideal in character themselves, that is, they have to do with vague but powerful conceptions of states of affairs that may be taken to be admirable in themselves. First among these reasons is the claim that human persons, though primarily moved by emotion and habit, are capable of episodic, contextual, and yet importantly self-defining uses of reason. We can and often do clarify, organize, and criticize our experience. When we do reason we make ourselves free or at least freer from the domination of the bad personal and social choices which often issue from the nonreflective and habitual expression of our emotions. And when we reason we do what is most characteristic of our species: We raise our conscious experience to self-consciousness and direct it accordingly. Embrace of the ideal of autonomous persons is a most appropriate way of underscoring and enhancing this unique human capacity to direct major portions of our experience with reason and in freedom. Embrace of the companion ideal of progressive societies, whose institutions are structured to protect and maximize the use of reason and freedom in social choosing, allows us to hope for an extension of practical personal autonomy to all members of our society and, in ideal, to all members of our species.

The second reason in the ideal for the choice of these specific ideals has to do with the ability of human persons and societies to transcend themselves, to go beyond the ideal and factual limitations imposed by any given state of reality. This ability is already implied in what has been said of reason and freedom; specifically, that beings capable of freely clarifying, organizing, and criticizing their experience are capable of going beyond its present limitations to a better future. This transcendence of fixed limitations is also implied in the bodies' physical evolution, in time and space consciousness, in the ability to store and share information outside the body, and especially in our powerful drives to discover facts and create ideals. This ability to transcend makes human persons and societies open in ideal to continued and indefinite progress. The ideals of autonomous persons in progressive societies allows for protection and enhancement of this human ability to transcend and thus fosters progress at the personal and social levels.

The first reason in fact for the choice of these ideals is an appeal to our intuitive morality and especially to our strongly felt "knowing" that an action or an institutional practice which is unjust to individual persons or to small groups would be wrong; wrong even if, at the same time, it maximizes the amount of happiness experienced by the greatest number of persons whose interest are involved. This moral intuition and others related to our use of the fundamental moral categories of good and bad, right and wrong are taken to be expressive of a nonreflective acknowledgment of the moral centrality of the human person. A theoretical account clarifying, organizing, and critically accepting these intuitions allows the formulation of an ethics of autonomy maximization, an ethics obviously consistent with the ideals of autonomous persons in progressive societies. This ethic directs us to first respect the human rights of all persons involved and then to do those actions and create those institutions which maximize, in order, practical personal autonomy, happiness, and pleasure.

The second factual claim in support of the ideals embraced here follows from an understanding that it is our societies and cultures which form the horizon against which persons and their moral intuitions are shaped. Thus the having of strong moral intuitions about the dignity of individual persons suggests the existence of social institutions and practices which, in however flawed a manner, tend to develop such intuitions in the persons whose habits these institutions and practices have helped to shape. In many contemporary societies, but especially in the democracies of the West, the prevailing religions, legal codes, and social conventions tend to protect and enhance personal dignity. If this is so, then the embrace of the ideals of autonomous persons in progressive societies is not utopian dreaming but the embrace of ideals which can in fact appeal meaningfully to persons in these societies. Thus, these ideals are eminently practical.

With these ideals in hand and with the tools of morality and an ethics to realize them, contemporary medicine and the personal and social realities associated with it can be profitably examined. Sickness is then seen not to be merely a source of pain and suffering, but also a compromise of this autonomy. Preservation and restoration of wellness is then primarily a preservation and restoration of practical personal autonomy. Concern for autonomy, along with concern for the prevention and palliation of pain and suffering, can be a meaningful and compassionate goal for contemporary medicine so long as there is an intelligent awareness of the consequent potential for blaming the sick inherent in an emphasis on personal responsibility in matters of sickness and well-being.

Protection and enhancement of practical personal autonomy is also a special part of the role of health care professionals in a complex society. Doctors, nurses, and all members of the health care professions are fiduciary agents who must act for the best interests of their patients. Awareness of this responsibility shows itself in clinical relationships in which a mutual participation model characterized by respect for patients' rights prevails. This is especially important in pediatric medicine where the patient cannot claim rights but must rely tacitly on the good will of others, and especially on that of the health care professional. Maximizing the number of doctors, nurses, and other members of the health care professions who spontaneously and habitually form such relationships with their patients requires that attention be paid to the moral character of medical education so that the health care providers of tomorrow are prepared for the challenges such relationships entail.

An understanding of this personal core of medical care must be part of the social dimensions of medicine where it is under enormous pressure in other directions. A stay in a modern hospital is for many patients an alienating and confusing experience just because this personal core of medicine is often overwhelmed there by economic, technological, and bureaucratic concerns. As we institutionalize our primary human relationships, so we define ourselves and the selves of our descendents. Consequently, we must insist on a hospital experience consistent with the ideals of autonomous persons in progressive societies. We must protect personal relationships in the hospital by defining and respecting patients' moral and legal rights and by taking steps to democratize the institutional structure of the hospital through increasing the range of participation by patients, potential patients, and the professionals who most intimately run the hospitals, nurses.

Another social dimension peculiar to medicine, and one which is morally troubling, is the need to use human subjects for medical experimentation. The use of human persons as subjects has been an important, perhaps indispensable, element in medicine's successes. If medicine is to continue to advance its ability to care for and cure persons in the future, experimentation with humans must continue to take place. Yet, as important a value as medical advance is, it cannot override our highest natural value, the human person. Therefore, research with human subjects must only be conducted under strict ethical guidelines insuring the protection of the subjects' human rights. Here as elsewhere, the maximization of the practical autonomy, happiness, and pleasure of persons can only be sought after the human rights of all those involved are secured.

A final social application of the ideals of autonomous persons in progressive societies looks to the future, to our growing powers to identify and predict genetically based and genetically related disease. A not unreasonable extrapolation of present genetic knowledge and power provides the promise and peril of near disease omniscience, the virtual ability to predict every person's future disease history, at least so far as that disease history is primarily genetic in cause. The promise is a future nearly free of genetic diseases and of the pain, suffering, and loss of autonomy which these diseases bring to persons' lives. The peril is a wholesale dehumanization of our reproductive lives and of the geneticist-patient relationship. Here again our ideals must dominate and direct these new facts. The rights of persons must be protected against mandatory genetic screening, mandatory sterilizations and abortions, and mandatory alterations in life-style. The health care professional relationship must preserve its fiduciary character: The best interests of the individual patient must prevail. And the collection, storage, and use of nearly omniscient genetic information must be subject to democratic political control. Thus we can insure that our new genetics is put under the control of persons, and that persons are not put under the control of the new genetics.

Throughout this book, the central general contention has been that the facts of medicine must be regulated by our ideals if we are to shape a reality which will be humanly better and whose facts will themselves be more open to shaping and reshaping by our ideals. It is appropriate that at the conclusion of this effort we anticipate and respond to some of the more obvious criticisms that can be brought against this central general contention.

Let us consider the simplist criticism first. It might be claimed that the numerous factual assertions made in the book are, some or many of them, not facts at all. It is especially likely that some will claim that it is just a cultural bias to assert that the western democracies are actually accommodating to the ideals we have described here. Of the general problem of the reliability of the facts asserted, it can only be said that these are the facts as they appear to me. It is the nature of assertions of fact that they are provisional and, where secure, the product of much human conversation and effort. If there are facts alleged here that are not facts, then the claim for them will at least be useful in calling out from others what truly are the facts or closer approximations of them. To the charge that the democracies of the West are not in fact as I have described them, I offer this thought experiment.[1] Presume for a moment that you espouse and hold dear the ideals of autonomous persons in progressive societies. Now presume that you could place yourself in any real human society, at any time now or in the past. There is only one condition. Having chosen your society and time, you have no control over what race, blood lineage, sex, ethnic group, or economic circumstances will be yours in that society at that time. In my case and in the cases of those with whom I have tried this experiment, choices of time and society seem to narrow quickly to contemporary societies identifying with the social achievements of the western democracies. Of course, this may simply be a way of clarifying and strengthening a cultural bias; but if so, it is a bias shaped by some significant facts about these societies.

It might also be claimed that the ideals offered here describe conceived states of affairs which are not admirable in themselves, or are too vague, or are misapplied to the facts. To the first charge, it can be admitted that there are indeed perspectives from which these ideals are not admirable ones. They have not always been taken to be so historically, and even when they came to be thought admirable by some they had to do intellectual, and sometimes real, combat with other ideals with which they are incompatible. So it may be that some will find these ideals uninviting. Nevertheless, they are put forth here with the hope that a significant and growing number of persons do find these ideals inherently admirable and that the reflective clarification, organization, and critical acceptance of them will itself increase that number. Furthermore, unlike the cases of many other incompatible ideals, the ideals of autonomous persons in progressive societies leave maximal room for harmonious co-existence with many other ideals, since they are, by their very natures, pluralistic in consequence. Of course, they are vague; ideals must be. Whether they are too vague or misapplied to the facts at hand must be left to the judgment of others; but again, left to others with the confidence that if there is something of importance here additional conversation and effort will tend to further determine these ideals and better apply them to fact.

It might be said by some that this whole work is far too relativistic, that it accept too easily the claim that there are other significant moral alternatives, and that it therefore provides no absolute foundation for the choice of these ideals and the associated ethical theory. In response, I admit to a good degree of relativism. It seems indisputable to me that other societies at other times have had different ideals and ethical codes than those offered here. The foundation I have tried to provide is the foundation of our human nature so far expressed, our human nature as historical and bodily beings. But history changes and the body has evolved. I consider it entirely possible that whole societies could still renounce completely the general ideals I have described here and do so with good will. I find it entirely possible that we could so alter our cultural and natural environments that even the most general features of human nature so far expressed could be changed. It is precisely because these ideals, this ethical theory, our received morality, and even human nature itself can be changed that reflection and personal commitment are now so very vital. We are, more so and faster than ever before, defining ourselves and the persons and societies of the future. And it is also because of this reality of change that progress is possible, not assured by any means, but possible. It relies on identification of the best ideals really available to us and action on our parts to realize these ideals in fact. There are no absolute foundations, therefore; but there are places to stand, viz., on the moral accomplishments of the past. F. H. Bradley made this point well.

> Morality is 'relative', but is none the less real. At every stage
> there is the social fact of the world so far moralized. There is
> an objective morality in the accomplished will of the past and
> present, a higher self worked out by the infinite pain, the sweat
> and blood of generations, and now given to me by free grace
> and in love and faith as a sacred trust.[2]

Finally, there is the possibility of one throughgoing criticism, the possibility of a wholesale rejection of the thesis that action on behalf of our ideals can change reality. This is the position of moral cynicism. To the moral cynic, reality is identical with the world of fact. It is a morally neutral battleground of egos and interests, a place where ideals are unimportant and irrelevant. If this is so, a major presumption of this book is

But these are abstract issues when one is dealing with medicine, which just is what it is because of the obvious efficacy of applying ideals to facts. Medicine stands out among human occupations for its intrinsic idealism, for the compassion for others that is and has been its animating spirit. Doctors, nurses, dentists, pharmacists, and the other members of the health care professions have as their controlling ideal, service to others in a most direct and intimate fashion. Medicine arises out of an attitude of caring for others, an attitude which is practically incompatible with moral cynicism. Furthermore, this is no romantic and idle caring, but a caring that directly engages the world of fact. Medicine is directed by its idealism, but is effective because it is empirical and has fashioned technologies for the care of persons.

Ironically, this very effectiveness of medicine has now so highlighted its relevance to fact and especially to cure that it has tended to obscure the ideals which have and ought to control these applications to fact and which have and ought to emphasize care. For many centuries, medicine had little to offer but idealism itself. Now, just as medicine has become a powerful technology for the factual improvement of human life and well-being, there are signs that that idealism is waning. It has been the intention of this book to reassert that idealism, to provide a conceptual framework, a vision, against which that traditional idealism can be articulated and used to control the new facts of medicine. Reality can be improved with this new medicine. It can be improved by increasing person's practical autonomy, by decreasing suffering and pain, and by doing so in a context of respect for persons' rights. The knowledge, the power, the professionals, and the institutions exist to do so, if we have the continuing will to do so. And above all, we shall need wisdom: the skill of interpreting the factual events of daily life in terms of an intelligent ideal worldview and of using this interpretation as the basis for making good decisions. We shall need such wisdom if we are to integrate ideal, fact, and medicine.
false, the presumption that ideals can make a difference in reality because reality is composed, in part, of our ideals. The first response to moral cynicism has to be that it appears to be false. Persons and societies certainly seem to be moved in events, great and small, not only by what they take to be the case in fact but also by what they take to be admirable in itself, that is, by their ideals. The cynic's rejoinder will likely be that this appearance is only that, an appearance. Morality, on the cynic's account, is only a rationalization for accomodation to blind fact, a masking of reality, a personal and social self-deception. Of course, this is an argument that cannot be decisively refuted. What can one say to a denial of what appears to be the case, except that it does indeed appear that way? But let us admit for a moment the possibility that the cynic is right, the possibility that belief in the efficacy of human ideals is self-deceptive. But let us also quickly add that it is equally possible that the cynic is the one who is deceived, the one whose selfishness, bitterness, or indolence is masking a genuine reality. There are no final rational means for determining who is right here. In such a rational impasse, it is fair to appeal to one other important dimension of our human experience: to our emotion laden will to

believe that our struggles on behalf of our ideals can make a difference and can therefore lend significance to our lives.[3] If we may both be self-deceived, then being self-deceived through belief in the importance of one's ideals is no worse in itself than being self-deceived through failure to believe in the importance of one's ideals — and belief has the additional advantages of accounting for the apparent facts and for the strongly felt emotion that our lives do have some significance. Finally, if the cynic is right, then nothing we do or say amounts to anything morally significant anyway; consequently, the cynic has no grounds on which to offer genuine criticism, since on this account nothing really matters at all.

CHAPTER 1
NOTES

1. For a general account of the nature of philosophy, see the entry "Philosophy" by John Passmore in the generally useful **Encyclopedia of Philosophy** by Paul Edwards (N.Y.: Macmillian and the Free Press, 1967). An interesting collection of essays which describe competing contemporary views of philosophy is **The Owl of Minera** ed. by Charles T. Bontempo and S. Jack Odell (N.Y.: McGraw-Hill, 1975).

2. This account of the logic of parts and wholes is influenced by Edmund Husserl's **Logical Investigations**, trans. by J. N. Findlay (N.Y.: Humanities Press, 1970).

3. This account of reality is drawn from the work of the American philosopher, Charles Sanders Peirce, and it depends on his scheme of categories. For Peirce, all wholes are triadic in structure. They are composed of a firstness element of pure possibility and freedom, a secondness element of resistance and contraint, and a thirdness element which integrates the other two elements under the headings of law and generality. In Peirce's terms, the conception of an ideal here is a first and that of a fact is a second. Reality, then, is the lawlike and general integration of ideal and fact. See **The Collected Papers of Charles S. Peirce** Vol I-VI ed. by Charles Hartshorne and Paul Weiss and vol. VII-VIII ed. by A. Burks (Cambridge: Harvard University Press, 1931, 1936, 1958). For an interpretation of Peirce's views on ideals, see **Charles S. Peirce on Norms and Ideals** by Vincent G. Potter, S.J. (Massachusetts: University of Massachusetts Press, 1967).

4. "There are some people - and I am one of them - who think that the most practical and important thing about a man is still his view of the universe. We think that for a landlady considering a lodger it is important to know his income, but still more important to know his philosophy." William James in **Pragmatism and Four Essays From the Meaning of Truth** ed. by Ralph Barton Perry (N.Y.: Meridian Books, 1955), p. 17.

5. A most influential contemporary reminder of the human dimensions of science is Thomas S. Kuhn's **The Structure of Scientific Revolutions** (Chicago: University of Chicago Press, 1970).

6. For elaboration of the need to proceed "as if" throughout a whole range of activities, see Hans Vaihinger, **The Philosophy of As If**, trans. by C. K. Ogden (N.Y. Harcourt, Brace, and Co., 1952).

7. For a general account of scientific theory, see Carl Hempel, **The Philosophy of the Natural Sciences** (New Jersey: Prentice-Hall, Inc., 1966).

8. See, for example, Peirce (Chapter 1, note 3) at 6.58-6.65; and **Nature and Life** by Alfred North Whitehead (Chicago: University of Chicago Press, 1938).

9. For an introduction to philosophy focused on ideals, see **Conflict of Ideals** by Luther J. Binkley (N.Y.: D. Van Nostrand Co., 1969). Anthropological and sociological literature is filled with treatments of ideals and their relationships to values and worldviews. See, for example, **Patterns of Culture** by Ruth Benedict (Cambridge: Riverside Press, 1959); **Variations In Value Orientation** by Florence R. Kluckhohn and Fred Strodtbeck (N.Y.: Ron, Peterson and Co., 1961); and **American Society: A Sociological Interpretation** by Robin Williams (N.Y.: Alfred A. Knopf, 1971).

10. For an application of this point to philosophy itself, see **Philosophy as Social Expression** by William Albert Levi (Chicago: University of Chicago Press, 1974).

11. On the "is-ought" problem generally, see **The Is-Ought Question** ed. by W. D. Hudson (London: Macmillan, 1969); and **The Is-Ought Problem: Its History, Analysis, and Dissolution** by W. M. Bruening (Washington, University Press of America, 1978).

12. On self-fulfilling commitments see William James' "The Sentiment of Rationality" and "The Will to Believe" in **William James Essays In Pragmatism** ed. by Alburey Castell (N.Y.: Hafner Press, 1948).

CHAPTER 2
NOTES

1. For the classical expression of this ideal, see Aristotle, **Nichomachean Ethics** trans. by Martin Ostwald (Indianapolis: The Liberal Arts Press, 1962).

2. Important twentieth century contributions to our appreciation of the emotional dimensions of morality were made by Charles L. Stevenson; see, for example, his article in **Mind,** "The Emotive Meaning of Ethical Terms," vol. 46, 1937. Also see A. J. Ayer's **Language Truth and Logic** (N.Y.: Dover Publications, Inc., 1952), esp. Chapter VI.

3. The ultimate intellectual satisfaction is to regard one's fundamental reasons or standards as being directly perceived, or directly grasped by the intelligence itself. See Aristotle, **Nichomachean Ethics** (op. cit. note 1), Book Six, especially at chapters 11 and 12.

4. For a sustained criticism of the idea of a mind separate from the larger person, see Gilbert Ryle, "Descartes' Myth" Chapter 1 of **The Concept of Mind** (N.Y.: Barnes and Noble, Inc., 1949).

5. See, for example, C.D. Broad, **Ethics and the History of Philosophy,** (London: Routledge and Kegan Paul, 1952), pp. 195-217; or Baruch Spinoza's Ethics, esp. Part II (Indianapolis: Hackett Publishing Company, 1982).

6. See, for example, C.A. Campbell's **In Defence of Free Will** (London: Allen and Unwin, 1967), pp. 27 ff.

7. On perfection see, for example, **The Perfectibility of Man** by John Passmore (N.Y.: Scribner Sons, 1971); also see Robert Nisbet's **History of the Idea of Progress** (N.Y.: Basic Books, 1980).

8. For a classic religious use of this point see St. Augustine's **Confessions** ed. by R.S. Pine-Coffin (N.Y.: Penguin Books, 1961).

9. This seems to be the heart of G.W.F. Hegel's Absolute Idealism. A secondary account of Hegel's system that focuses on God is Quentin Lauer's **Hegel's Concept of God** (Albany: State University of New York Press, 1982).

CHAPTER 3
NOTES

1. For perspectives on the human rights picture worldwide, see **Human Rights** ed. by Thomas Draper (N.Y.: The H.W. Wilson Co., 1982). Also see **Basic Rights** by Henry Shue (Princeton: Princeton University Press, 1980); and **The Philosophy of Human Rights** ed. by Alan S. Rosenbaum (Connecticut: Greenwood Press, 1980).

2. The following account of the self is influenced by the contributions of the existentialists, esp. Heidegger, Sartre, and Camus. For introductory accounts of this school of thought, see **Existentialism** by Mary Warnock (London: Oxford University Press, 1970); **The Existentialists, A Critical Study** by James D. Collins (Chicago: H. Regnery Co., 1952); and **An Existentialist Ethics** by Hazel Barnes (N.Y.: Alfred H. Knopf, 1967).

3. **Being and Time,** Martin Heiddegger, trans. by John Marquarrie and Edward Robinson (N.Y.: Harper and Row, 1962), esp. Division Two, I on "Being-Towards-Death."

4. See, for example, **Existentalism and Human Emotions** by J.P. Sartre (N.Y.: Philosophical Library, 1957).

5. On the self's creation of value, see generally, **The Myth of Sisyphus and Other Essays** by Albert Camus (N.Y.: Alfred A. Knopf, Inc., 1955); or any of Friedrich Nietzsche's works.

6. See Aristotle on the relationship between self-love and friendship (Chapter 2, note 1), pp. 260-263.

7. The following discussion of the social dimensions of the self is indebted to **Mind, Self, and Society** by George Herbert Mead (Chicago: University of Chicago Press, 1962); and to **The World and the Individual** by Josiah Royce, (N.Y.: Macmillan Company, 1901).

8. To learn a language is to enter into a "form of life." See Ludwig Wittgenstein, **Philosophical Investigations** trans. by G.M. Anscombe (N.Y.: Macmillan Company, 1968) esp. numbers 19, 23, and 241.

9. The claim that there is an analogy between self and society is at least as old as Plato's **Republic,** Book I, in **Plato, The Collected Dialogues,** ed. by Edith Hamilton and Huntington Cairns (New Jersey: Princeton University Press, 1969).

10. Here and throughout this work, references to the significance of democracy reflect the influence of the works of John Dewey. For an introductory sample of Dewey's contributions, see **The Moral Writings of John Dewey** ed. by James Gouinlock (N.Y.: Hafner Press, 1976).

11. "Beings whose existence depends not on our will but on nature have, nevertheless, if they are not rational beings, only a relative value as means and are therefore called things. On the other hand, rational beings are called persons inasmuch as their nature already marks them out as ends in themselves, i.e., as something which is not to be used merely as means and hence there is imposed thereby a limit on all arbitrary use of such beings, which are thus objects of respect." Immanuel Kant **Grounding for the Metaphysics of Morals** trans. by James W. Ellington (Indianapolis: Hackett Publishing Co., 1981), pp. 35-36.

12. See, for example, **On Being A Christian** by Hans Kung, trans. by Edward Quinn, (N.Y.: Doubleday, 1976).

13. See, for example, **The Concept of Law** by H.L.A. Hart (Oxford: Oxford University Press, 1961).

14. The ideal of civility in the West was clearly stated by Aristotle, again see the **Nichomachean Ethics** at Book Four. Institutional aid to the needy in the context of liberal democracy is given a persuasive justification by John Rawls in **A Theory of Justice** (Cambridge: Harvard University Press, 1971). The classic statement of the value of individuality in western democracies is in **On Liberty** by John Stuart Mill, (Indianapolis: Hackett Publishing Co., 1978) esp. Chapter III, pp. 53-71.

15. See, for example, Louis Henkin, **The Rights of Man Today** (Colorado: Westview Press, 1978).

16. A useful compendium of contemporary statements dealing with human rights in a variety of contexts is **Basic Documents on Human Rights** ed. by Ian Brownlie, (Oxford: Claredon Press, 1981).

17. Recent philosophical accounts of negative and positive rights include **Philosophy and Public Policy** by Sidney Hook (Carbondale: Illinois University Press, 1980); and **Rights and Persons** by A.I. Melden (Berkeley: University of California Press, 1977).

CHAPTER 4
NOTES

1. An influence here is the metaethical school of intuitionists, esp. the work of G.E. Moore. See his **Principia Ethica** (Cambridge: Cambridge University Press, 1968). Also see H.A. Pritchard "Does Moral Philosophy Rest on a Mistake" in **Readings In Ethical Theory** ed. by Wilfrid Sellars and John Hospers (New Jersey: Prentice-Hall, Inc., 1970).

2. On the importance of the context of learning for the understanding of a concept's meaning, see Wittgenstein (Chapter 1, note 8), esp. at 190, 197, 362, and 556.

3. This discussion of the unique and the similar in morality, as well as much of the following discussion of ethics in general is indebted to William Frankena's **Ethics** (New Jersey: Prentice-Hall, Inc., 1973). For an existential account of moral uniqueness see J.P. Sartre (Chapter 3, note 4) pp. 24 and following.

4. Language then would be wholly private and a private language is no language at all. Again, consult Wittgenstein (Chapter 1, note 8) esp. at 268, 275, and the discussion which follows.

5. For a general introduction to issues in contemporary philosophy of language, see **The Underlying Reality of Language** by Jerrold J. Katz (N.Y.: Harper & Row, 1971).

6. For discussions of the prescriptive force of morality, see R. M. Hare, **The Language of Morals** (N.Y.: Oxford University Press, 1964); and **Freedom and Reason** (Oxford: Clarendon Press, 1963).

7. The classical description of weakness of the will is Aristotle's. See **Nichomachean Ethics** (Chapter 2, note 1), Book Seven.

8. See Peirce (Chapter 1, note 3) at 5.377 and following for insight into the strengths and weaknesses of the "method of tenacity."

CHAPTER 5
NOTES

1. On the remarkable phenomenon of self-desception, see Herbert Fingarette's **Self-deception** (N.Y.: Humanities Press, 1969).

2. See, for example, **The Existence of God** ed. by John Hick (N.Y.: Macmillan Co., 1963); and **Does God Exist?** by Hans Kung, trans. by Edward Quinn (N.Y.: Vintage Books, 1981).

3. Indeed, the first person in the western philosophical tradition to apply ethical criticism to a conventional morality was put to death for his efforts. See, **The Last Days of Socrates** (a collection of Plato's Socratic dialogues) trans. and ed. by Hugh Tredennick (Baltimore: Penguin Books, 1974).

4. This is St. Thomas Aquinas' formulation. See, **Summa Theologica** (N.Y.: Benziger, 1947) at I-IIae, Q. 94.

5. The classical statement of utilitarianism is J.S. Mill's **Utilitarianism** ed. by Samuel Gorovitz (Indianapolis: Bobbs-Merrill, 1971). Recent examinations of the theory include **Forms and Limits of Utilitarianism** by David Lyons (Oxford: Clarendon Press, 1965); **Utilitarianism, For and Against** ed. by J.J.C. Smart and B. Williams (Cambridge: Cambridge University Press, 1973); and **Utilitarianism and Beyond** ed. by Amartya Sen (Cambridge: Cambridge University Press, 1982).

6. Jeremy Bentham, the founder of utilitarianism, was a leader in early nineteenth century efforts to reform and democratize the British Parliament. See, for example, **Bentham** by James Steintrager (Ithaca, N.Y.: Cornell University Press, 1977). A generation later, John Stuart Mill used the principles of utilitarianism to champion the liberation of women and to condem racial slavery and the oppression of the Irish. See, Michael St. John Packe, **The Life of John Stuart Mill** (London: Secker and Warburg, 1954). Contemporary utilitarians have used the principle similarly; for example, to call for a more just worldwide distribution of wealth and to condemn our treatment of animals. See, for example, **Practical Ethics** by Peter Singer (Cambridge, U.K.; Cambridge University Press, 1979).

7. J.S. Mill writes that even some of the most esteemed minds regarded those who support the view that a human life has no higher end than pleasure as holding "a doctrine worthy only of swine. . . ." **Utilitarianism** (op. cit., note 6) Chapter II.

8. This distance is less if the principle of utility is applied to moral rules and not to individual acts, but I am presuming that such a distinction

between "rule" and "act" utilitarianism is not ultimately tenable. On this point, see Smart's discussion at pp. 9-12 in his work with Williams (**op. cit.**, note 5). The possibility of holding either a pure act or pure rule position of any kind is incompatible with the need to recognize both the morally unique and the morally similar; see above Chapter 4, B.

9. See, for example, Charles J. Dougherty and Vern R. Walker, "Scientific Medicine, Technology, and the Concept of Health," **Ethics In Science and Medicine**, vol. 5, pp. 75-81.

10. For a more extended discussion of the wrongfulness of harming persons, see **Right and Wrong** by Charles Fried (Cambridge: Harvard University Press, 1978).

11. There are ancient and biblical antecedents to the notion of rights; see Henkin, **The Rights of Man Today** (Chapter 3, note 15). The case for the importance of natural law theory in the Christian medieval philosophers as the historical underpinning for the rise of the modern idea of rights is made by Jacques Maritain in **The Rights of Man and Natural Law**, trans. by Doris Anson, (N.Y.: Scribner's Sons, 1943); and by A. Passerin d'Entreves in **The Medieval Constrition to Political Thought** (London, Oxford University Press, 1939).

12. Martin P. Golding, "The Concept of Rights: A Historical Sketch" in **Bioethics and Human Rights** ed. by E. Bandman and B. Bandman (Boston: Little, Brown and Company, 1978), p. 44-50.

13. See, for example, R. Forster and J. Greene, ed. of **Preconditons of Revolution In Early Modern Europe** (Baltimore: John Hopkins Press, 1970); L. Krieger, **Kings and Philosophers** (N.Y.: W.W. Norton, 1970); and R. Palmer, **The Age of Democratic Revolutions** (Princeton: Princeton University Press, 1964).

CHAPTER 6
NOTES

1. The argument of this section follows that of Immanuel Kant's **Grounding for the Metaphysics of Morals** (Chapter 3, note 11).

2. For an interesting exploration of this, see Thomas Nagel's "Moral Luck" in his **Mortal Questions** (Cambridge: Cambridge University Press, 1979).

3. On the subjectivity of such choices, see Soren Kierkegaard's "Truth Is Subjectivity" in **A Kierkegaard Anthology** ed. by Robert Bretall (N.Y.: The Modern Library, 1946), p. 210 and following.

4. **Op. cit.**, Kant, pp. 26 and 30.

5. See, for example, Sissela Bok's **Lying** (N.Y.: Vintage Books, 1979), p. 98.

6. The allusion, of course, is to Friedrich Nietzsche; see his **Beyond Good and Evil** trans. by Helen Zimmern, vol. 12, **The Complete Works of Friedrich Nietzsche** (N.Y.: Russell and Russell, 1964).

7. Aristotle displays the cultural limitations of even the most acute of thinkers when he suggests that only free and socially equal males are capable of genuine friendship. See **Nichomachean Ethics** (Chapter 2, note 1) at Book Eight.

8. The abortion debate has produced several criteria of being a person, criteria offered specifically to exclude the fetus. Mary Anne Warren in "On the Moral and Legal Status of Abortion," **Monist**, vol. 57, no. 1, 1973 claims a human must have at least one of the following characteristics to be a person with rights: consciousness, reasoning, self-motivated activity, capacity to communicate, or self-concepts and self-awareness. In a striking moment of candor, she ends a postscript to her article with this: ". . . it follows from my argument that when an unwanted or defective infant is born into a society which cannot afford and/or is not willing to care for it, then its destruction is permissible." Joseph Flectcher in **The Ethics of Genetic Control** (N.Y.: Doubleday, 1974), p. 137, offers the view that ". . . perhaps something like a score of 20 on the Binet scale of I.Q. would be roughly but realistically a minimum or base line for personal status."

9. This is what St. Thomas Aquinas called "invincible ignorance." See **Summa Theologica** (Chapter 5, note 4) at I-IIae, Q. 76.

10. On the nature of special rights, see H. L. A. Hart, "Are There Any Natural Rights," **Philosophical Review**, vol. 64, 1955, p. 183; and

Sidney Hook (Chapter 3, note 17) at p. 75; and A. I. Mellen (Chapter 3, note 17) at p. 56.

11. This dialectic of the self and others is explored in Josiah Royce's **Philosophy of Loyalty** (N.Y.: Macmillan Co., 1908) and its application to Christianity made clear in his **The Problem of Christianity** (N.Y.: Macmillan Co., 1913).

12. "Growth itself is the only moral 'end'." John Dewey, **Reconstruction In Philosophy** (Boston: Beacon press, 1957), p. 117.

13. See, for example, Christopher Lasch, **The Culture of Narcissism** (N.Y.: Norton, 1978).

CHAPTER 7
NOTES

1. For a penetrating analysis of bodily consciousness consult **The Phenomenology of Perception** by Maurice Merleau-Ponty (London: Routledge and Kegan Paul Ltd., 1962).

2. Peirce sees the consciousness of being wrong as a fundamental episode in the genesis of self-consciousness. See, **The Collected Papers of Charles Sanders Peirce** (Chapter 1, note 3) at 5.233.

3. For a general account of the connection between sickness, health, and personal autonomy, see H. Tristram Engelhardt Jr., "Human Well-Being and Medicine: Some Basic Value Judgments in the Biomedical Sciences," in **Science, Ethics and Medicine,** ed. by H. Tristram Engelhardt Jr. and Daniel Callahan, (N.Y.: Hastings Center, 1976) esp. pp. 124-127.

4. "In the field of psychiatry, the central question about human conduct in general thus remains what it has always been, namely, **the meaning of human autonomy.**" Stephen Toulmin, "Introductory Note: The Multiple Aspects of Mental Health and Mental Disorder," **Journal of Medicine and Philosophy,** vol. 2, no. 3, 1977, p. 194.

5. An excellent study of this phenomenon is **The Denial of Death** by Ernest Becker (N.Y.: Macmillan, 1973).

6. The full W.H.O. statement can be found in "Preamble to the Constitution of the World Health Organization," **The First Ten Years of the World Health Organization** (Geneva: World Health Organization, 1958). The analysis which follows here is indebted to Daniel Callahan, "The WHO Definition of Health," **Hastings Center Studies,** vol. 1, no. 3, 1973, p. 77-87.

7. "In its strict sense, 'health' refers to individual organisms — plants and animals, no less than humans — and only, analogously or metaphysically to large groupings." Leon R. Kass, "Regarding the End of Medicine and the Pursuit of Health," **The Public Interest,** no. 40, Summer 1975, p. 19.

8. See "Soviet Psychiatry on Trial; Vote of the World Psychiatric Association" by W. Reich, **Commentary,** vol. 65, January 1978, pp. 40-48; and "Political Prisoners in the Psychiatric Ward" by F. Willey, et. al., **Newsweek,** vol. 99, January 11, 1982, pp. 31-32.

9. See, for example, Stephen R. Kellert, "A Sociocultural Concept of Health and Illness," **Journal of Philosophy and Medicine** vol. 1, no. 3, 1976, esp. at p. 222.

10. See, for example, Sissela Bok "The Ethics of Giving Placebos," **Scientific American** vol. 231, 1974, pp. 17-23.

11. For discussions of human attitudes toward diseases of animals and plants, see Peter Sedgwick, "Illness-Mental and Otherwise," **Hastings Center Studies,** vol. 1, no. 3, 1973, p. 30; and H. Tristram Engelhardt Jr., "Ideology and Etiology," **Journal of Medicine and Philosophy,** vol. 1, no. 3, 1976, p. 264.

12. The classic description of the sick role is contained in **The Social System** by Talcott Parsons (N.Y.: Free Press, 1951), pp. 428-73. Also, see Miriam Siegler and Humphrey Oswald, "The 'Sick Role' Revisited," **Hastings Center Studies,** vol. 1, no. 3, 1973.

13. See, for example, Robert M. Veatch, "Who Should Pay for Smokers' Medical Care" **Hastings Center Report,** vol. 4, 1974, p. 8-9.

14. See, for example, Warren F. Gorman, "Malingering," **Arizona Medicine,** Vol. XXXVIII, no. 8, August, 1981, pp 616-618.

15. Indeed, some have raised doubts about the category of mental illness itself; see, **The Myth of Mental Illness** by Thomas S. Szasz (N.Y.: Doubleday and Co., 1961).

16. See, for example, Barbara and John Ehrenreich, "The American Health Empire: The System Behind the Chaos," in their **American Health Empire: Power, Profits, and Politics** (N.Y.: Random House, 1970).

17. On access to emergency care, see Charles J. Dougherty, "The Right to Health Care: First Aid in the Emergency Room," **Public Law Forum,** vol. 4, no. 1, 1984, pp. 101-128.

CHAPTER 8
NOTES

1. From the **New York Times Magazine**, May 23, 1982, p. 24: "According to the most recent figures available the average doctor earns $79,700 per year . . . . The average surgeon earns a little more: according to the 1979 figures, at 35 he or she earned $77,800; between 36 and 40, $99,700; between 41 and 45, $112,400; and a little over $100,000 between 46 and 60.

2. For a fuller discussion of the moral dimensions of being a professional, see **The Moral Foundations of Professional Ethics** by Alan H. Goldman, (N.J.: Rowman and Littlefield, 1980).

3. "The core of the physician's obligation under the law of medical malpractice lies in the statement that he must employ such reasonable skill and care as are commonly exercised by average reputable physicians in the same general line or school of practice in the same locality or in localities substantially similar to it." **Cases and Materials on Law and Medicine** by Walter Wadlington, Jon R. Waltz, and Roger B. Dworkin (N.Y.: Foundation Press, 1980), p. 322.

4. See, for example, A.R. Jonsen, "Do No Harm" **Annals of Internal Medicine,** vol. 88, 1978, pp. 827-832; and by the same author, "History of Medical Ethics" in **Encyclopedia of Bioethics** (N.Y.: Free Press, 1978), pp. 567-570. For an opposing view, consult L.J. Nelson, "Primum Utilis Esse: The Primacy of Usefulness in Medicine," **Yale Journal of Biology and Medicine,** vol. 51, 1978, pp. 655-667.

5. See, for example, Zeev Ben-Sira, "The Foundation of the Professional's Affective Behavior in Client Satisfaction: A Revised Approach to Social Interaction Theory," **Journal of Health and Social Behavior,** vol. 17, March, 1976, pp. 3-11; and B. Hulka, et al. "Communication, Compliance, and Concordance betwen Physicians and Patients With Prescribed Medications," **American Journal of Public Health,** vol. 67, 1977, p. 847 and ff.

6. **The Law of Medical Malpractice** by Joseph H. King, Jr. (St. Paul, Minnesota: West Publishing Co., 1977), pp. 8-35.

7. For a further discussion of this right in the medical context, see Alexander M. Capron, "A Functional Approach to Informed Consent," **University of Pennsylvania Law Review,** vol. 123, December 1974, pp. 364-371.

8. See, for example, Franz J. Ingelfinger, "Informed (But Uneducated) Consent," **The New England Journal of Medicine,** vol. 287, August, 1972, pp. 465-466.

9. This account of the doctor-patient relationship is based on my "Moral Directionality in the Doctor-Patient Relationship," **Linacre Quarterly**, vol. 44, no. 4, 1977, pp. 361-367. That account is itself indebted to T. Szasz and M. Hollender, "The Basic Models of the Doctor-Patient Relationship," **Archives of Internal Medicine**, vol. 97, May, 1969, p. 585 ff.; and to R. Veatch, "Models for Ethical Medicine in a Revolutionary Age," **Hastings Center Report**, vol. 2, no. 3, June, 1972, p. 5 and ff.

10. See, for example, B. Korsch and V. Negrete, "Doctor-Patient Communication," **Scientific American**, August, 1972, p. 66.

11. Sissela Bok describes the following benefits of fully informing patients of their conditions. "Pain is tolerated more easily, recovery from surgery is quicker, and cooperation with therapy is greatly improved." **Lying**, (Chapter 6, note 5), p. 247.

12. **Op. cit.**, Ben-Sira, note 5.

13. A graphic, if overstated, account of the causes for this alienation can be found in **Medical Nemesis** by Ivan Illich (N.Y.: Pantheon Press, 1976).

14. An interesting popular account of contemporary medical education appeared in **The New York Times Magazine**, May 23 and 30, 1982. The article, "The Making of a Doctor" by David Black ends with this concern: "If medical education does not come to grips with the ethical as well as the technical changes in the field, society may soon discover that modern medicine has given a relatively small number of men and women enormous power - which they have not been adequately trained to wield."

15. The most influential recent account of hospital dying is **On Death and Dying** by Elizabeth Kubler-Ross (N.Y.: Macmillan Co., 1969).

16. See, for example, **Autonomous Technology** by Langdon Winner (Cambridge: MIT Press, 1977).

17. See John Dewey's perceptive views on the teaching of science in his **Democracy and Education** (N.Y.: Free Press, 1966), pp. 219-230.

18. Nurses also have special educational needs having to do with their professional relationships with physicians, a relationship often soured by sexism. On this issue, see E. Joy Kroeger Mappes, "Ethical Dilemmas for Nurses: Physicians' Orders versus Patients' Rights" in **Biomedical Ethics**, ed. by T. Mappes and J. Zembaty (N.Y.: McGraw-Hill Book Co., 1981) pp. 95-102.

CHAPTER 9
NOTES

1. There is a growing literature on children's rights. Recent works include **Children's Rights** ed. by Patricia Vardin and Ilene Brady (N.Y.: Teachers College Press, 1979); **Birthrights** by Richard Farson (N.Y.: Penguin Books, 1978); **Equal Rights for Children** by Howard Cohen (New Jersey: Rowman and Littlefield, 1980); and **The Rights of Children** ed. by Albert E. Wilkenson (Philadelphia: Temple University Press, 1973).

2. Contemporary discussions of rights connect them intimately with the ability to claim; see, for example, Joel Feinberg, "The Nature and Value of Rights," **The Journal of Value Inquiry,** vol. 4, 1970, pp. 243-257.

3. Thus Principle 2 of the United Nations' "Declaration of the Rights of the Child" asserts that the child has rights to "enjoy special protection" and the opportunities ". . . to develop physically, mentally, morally, spiritually and socially in a healthy and normal manner and in conditions of freedom and dignity." See U.N. General Assembly Resolution 1386 (XIV), November 20, 1959, in **Official Records of the General Assembly,** Fourteenth Session, Supp. no. 16, 1960, pp. 19 ff.

4. For an interesting discussion of the moral foundations of parental proxy consent, see Richard McCormick, "Proxy Consent in the Experimentation Situation," **Perspectives in Biology and Medicine,** vol. 18, no. 1, August, 1974, pp. 2-20.

5. See, for example, "Problems In Defining Child Abuse and Neglect" by Natalie Abrams and "Foster Care - In Whose Best Interest" by Robert H. Mnooklin, both of which are in **Having Children** ed. by Onora O'Neill and William Ruddick (N.Y.: Oxford University Press, 1979) at pp. 156 and 179 respectively.

6. See, for examples, D. S. Burgess, "An International Perspective on Children's Rights" in **Children's Rights,** (op. cit., note 1), p. 112.

7. E.E. Werner, **Cross-Cultural Child Development** (California: Brooks/Cole Publishing, 1979), p. 53.

8. For recent work in child development, see **Childhood: The Study of Development** by Robert Leve (N.Y.: Random House, 1980); and **Child Development and Personality** by Paul Henry Mussen, John J. Couger, and Jerome Kagan (N.Y.: Harper & Row, 1979).

9. See, for example, P. Blos, "Children Think About Illness: Their Concepts and Beliefs," in **Psychosocial Aspects of Pediatric Care,** ed. by E. Gellert (N.Y.: Harcourt, Brace, Jovanovich, 1978), p. 12 and ff.

10. For more on the world of the child consult the important work of Jean Piaget in **The Essential Piaget** ed. by Howard E. Guber and J. Jacque Voneche (N.Y.: Basic Books, 1977).

11. For a specific discussion of some of these issues, see N. Frost, "Ethical Problems in Pediatrics," in **Current Problems in Pediatrics,** vol. VI, no. 12, October, 1976, p. 27 ff.

12. An overview of some of the modern technologies available to psychiatry is contained in **Behavior Control** by Perry London (N.Y.: New American Library, 1977).

13. See, for example, Robert M. Veatch, "Choosing Not to Prolong Dying," **Medical Dimensions,** December, 1972. Also, Richard McCormick has developed guidelines for allowing radically defective infants to die, guidelines which would be applicable in the cases of dying adults as well: "To Save or Let Die: The Dilemma of Modern Medicine," **Journal of the American Medical Association,** vol. 229, July, 1974, pp. 172-176.

14. See Paul Ramsey, "On (Only) Caring for the Dying," Chapter 3 of **Patient as Person** (New Haven: Yale University Press, 1970), esp. pp. 153-157.

CHAPTER 10
NOTES

1. For accounts of the nature of democracy see **Democratic Political Theory** by J. Roland Pennock (Princeton: Princeton University Press, 1979); **The Life and Times of Liberal Democracy** by C. B. MacPherson (Oxford: Oxford University Press, 1977); and **Democracy and Illusion** by John Plamenatz (London: Longman Group Limited, 1973).

2. For a discussion of the translation of moral rights into legal rights, see **Taking Rights Seriously** by Ronald Dworkin (Cambridge: Harvard University Press, 1977), esp. the chapter of the same name.

3. "Full education comes only when here is a responsible share on the part of each person, in proportion to capacity, in shaping the aims and the policies of the social groups to which he belongs. This fact fixes the significance of democracy." John Dewey **Reconstruction In Philosophy** (Chapter 6, note 13), p. 209.

4. The average American is hospitalized eleven times before his or her death. See **The Rights of Hospital Patients** by George J. Annas (N.Y.: Avon Books, 1975), p. 1.

5. See, eg., Eli Ginsberg, "The Monetarization of Medical Care," **New England Journal of Medicine,** vol. 310, no. 18; Paul Starr, **The Social Transformation of American Medicine** (N.Y.: Basic Books, 1982), esp. pp. 430-436; and A. Relman, "Investor-Owned Hospitals and Health-Care Costs," **New England Journal of Medicine,** vol. 309, no. 6, pp. 370-372.

6. See, for example, Charles J. Dougherty and Vern R. Walker, "Scientific Medicine, Technology, and the Concept of Health," (Chapter 5, note 9).

7. This discussion of hospital patients' legal rights is based on Charles J. Dougherty and Sandra L. Dougherty, "Moral Reconstruction In The Hospital: A Legal and Philosophical Perspective on Patient Rights," **Creighton Law Review,** vol. 14, no. 4 (supp.), 1981.

8. 54 Del. 15, 174 A.2d 135 (1961).

9. Mercy Medical Center of Oshkosh, Inc. v. Winnebago County, 58 Wis.2d 260, —, 206 N.W.2d 198, 201 (1973).

10. Guerrero v. Cooper Queen Hospital, 112 Ariz. 104, —, 537, P.2d 1329, 1331 (1975).

11. 211 N.Y. 125, 105 N.E. 92 (1914).

12. Sard v. Hardy, 281 Md. 432, —, 379 A.2d 1014, 1020 (1977).

13. Canterbury v. Spence, 464 F.2d 772, 778-79 (D.C. Cir. 1972).

14. See, for example, Warner v. Taylor, 272 N.C. 386, —, 158 S.E.2d 339, 344 (1968).

15. See both Sard v. Hardy and Canterbury v. Spence, notes 12 and 13 above.

16. Op. cit., Annas, p. 117.

17. These decisions, respectively, are: Pyramid Life Insurance v. Masonic Hospital Association of Payne County, 191 F. Supp. 51, 54 (W.D. Okla. 1961) and Gotkin v. Miller, 514 F.2d 125 (2d Cir. 1975).

18. For example, see Community Hospital Association v. District Court in and for Boulder County, 194 Colo. 98, 570 P.2d 243 (1977).

19. **Op. cit.**, Annas, p. 123.

20. A. Cantor, "A Patient's Decision to Decline Life-Saving Medical Treatment: Bodily Integrity versus the Preservation of Life," **Rutgers Law Review,** vol. 26, p. 228, 1973.

21. Application of President and Directors of Georgetown College, Inc., 331 F.2d 1000 (D.C. Cir.), **cert. den.,** 377 U.S. 978 (1964); United States v. George, 239 F. Supp. 752 (D. Conn. 1965); John F. Kennedy Memorial Hospital v. Heston, 58 N.J. 576, 279 A.2d 670 (1971).

22. 32 Ill. 2d 361, 205 N.E.2d 435 (1965).

23. See, for example, In re Quinlan, 70 N.J. 10, 355 A.2d 647 (1976).

24. 373 Mass. 728, 370 N.E.2d 417 (1977).

25. — Mass. —, 393 N.E.2d 836 (1979).

26. See generally, Comment, "The Action of Abandonment in Medical Malpractice Litigation," **Tulane Law Review,** vol. 36, 834, 1962.

27. Bedard v. Notre Dame Hospital, 89 R.I. 195, 151 A.2d 690 (1959).

28. A useful overview of grounds for litigation in this area is available in **The Law of Medical Malpractice** by Joseph H. King, Jr., Chapter 8, note 6.

29. For contemporary philosophical discussions of this issue see the entire volume of **Journal of Medicine and Philosophy,** vol. 4, 1979.

30. U.N. Doc. A/810, December 10, 1948.

31. **Op. cit.**, Annas, p. 178.

32. The claim that need is the most appropriate basis on which to distribute health care (as opposed to merit, contribution to society, or money) is developed by Gene Outka, "Social Justice and Equal Access to Health Care," **Journal of Religious Ethics**, vol. 2, no. 1, Spring, 1974.

33. For a perspective on nurses and their advocacy for patients, see Elsie Bandman, "The Rights of Nurses and Patients: A Case for Advocacy," in **Bioethics and Human Rights** (Chapter 8, note 18), p. 332-338.

CHAPTER 11
NOTES

1. Slowing the rate of medical progress is something we can afford, but undermining the moral basis of society is something we can not. For the development of this point, see Hans Jonas, "Philosophical Reflections on Experimenting with Human Subjects," **Experimentation With Human Subjects,** ed. by Paul A. Freund (N.Y.: George Braziller, 1969).

2. Documentation of these cases can be found in Henry K. Beecher, "Ethics and Clinical Research," **The New England Journal of Medicine,** vol. 274, 1966, pp. 1354-60; in Robert M. Veatch and Sharmon Sollitto, "Human Experimentation —The Ethical Questions Persist," **The Hastings Center Report,** vol. 3, no. 3, June, 1973; and in Alexander M. Capron, "Medical Research In Prisons" in that same **Hastings Center Report.**

3. This case is discussed in some detail by Paul Ramsey in his **Patient as Person** esp. at pp. 53-54 (see note 14, Chapter 9).

4. The source for this discussion of Nazi medical experimentation is Leo Alexander, "Medical Science Under Dictatorship," **New England Journal of Medicine,** vol. 241, 1949, pp. 39-47.

5. This view is held by Paul Ramsey. See his "Consent as a Canon of Loyalty with Special Reference to Children in Medical Investigation" in **Patient as Person** (note 14, Chapter 9).

6. For a general treatment of experimentation in the prison context, see Jessica Mitford, **Kind and Usual Punishment,** (N.Y.: Alfred A. Knopf, Inc., 1972).

7. For a study of such experiments, see Arthur Schafer, "The Ethics of the Randomized Clinical Trial," **The New England Journal of Medicine,** vol. 307, no. 12, 1982, pp. 719-724.

8. For a discusssion of paying research subjects, consult Marx Wartofsky, "On Doing It For Money," **National Commission for the Protection of Human Subjects of Biomedical and Behavior Research,** 1976. DHEW Publication No. (OS) 76-132.

9. Perhaps the most comprehensive general discussion of these issues is to be found in **Experimentation with Human Beings,** by Jay Katz (N.Y.: Russell Sage Foundation, 1973).

10. For the text of the Nuremberg Code, see United States v. Karl Brandt, et. al., **Trials of War Criminals Before Nuremberg Military Tribunals Under Control Council Law No. 10,** (October, 1946 - April, 1949).

CHAPTER 12
NOTES

1. For an overview of some of what is already the case, see Tabitha M. Powledge, "Genetic Screening," **Encyclopedia of Bioethics**, ed. by Warren T. Reich (N.Y.: Free Press, 1978, pp. 567-572.

2. The use of such biomarkers in the prediction and early detection of cancer is discussed in **Biomarkers In Hereditary Cancer**, ed. by Henry T. Lynch and Hoda Guirgus (N.Y.: Van Nostrand Reinhold, forthcoming).

3. A general treatment of the control of the new genetics within a democratic political framework is provided in **The Political Implications of Human Genetic Technology**, by R.H. Blank (Colorado: Westview Press, 1981).

4. See John A. Osmundsen, "We Are All Mutants - Preventive Genetic Medicine: A Growing Clinical Field Troubled by a Confusion of Ethics," **Medical Dimensions**, Febraury, 1973, p. 6.

5. Charles Fried in "The Lawyer As Friend: The Moral Foundations of the Lawyer-Client Relationship," **Yale Law Journal**, vol. 85, 1976, p. 1060 ff. makes a similar claim in a defense of the personal core of the lawyer-client relationship. "For it is just the point about emergencies and wars that they create special, brutal, and depersonalized relations which civilization, by its very essence, must keep from becoming the general rule of social life." (p. 1077). See also **Triage and Justice** by Gerald R. Winston (Berkeley: University of California Press, 1982).

6. For a different view see **The Ethics of Genetic Control** by Joseph Fletcher (Chapter 6, note 9), esp. pp. 182-3. Though admitting that voluntary screening would be "nicer," Fletcher urges us to ". . .let it be compulsory if need be, for the common good. . . ." He then describes a "socially conscientious system" of national registry of genetic information: skin and blood tests of all infants, computer storage of the genetic information gleaned, and examination of the genetic compatibilities of all applicants for marriage licenses.

7. See Sissela Bok's **Lying**, Chapter XV, "Lies to the Sick and Dying," (Chapter 6, note 5).

8. For a treatment of the hazards of the idea of seeking genetic perfection in fact, consult Daniel Callahan, "The Meaning and Significance of Genetic Disease," **Ethical Issues In Human Genetics: Genetic Counseling and the Use of Genetic Knowledge**, ed. by Bruce Hilton, et. al., (New York: Phenum Publishing Corporation, 1973), pp.

83-90. Also see the article by Leon R. Kass, "Implications of Prenatal Diagnosis for the Human Right to Life," in that same volume.

9. See, for example, M.A. Stenchever, "An Abuse of Prenatal Diagnosis" (letter to the editor), **Journal of the American Medical Association,** vol. 221, 1972, p. 408.

10. See, for example, Rene Dubos' **Mirage of Health,** (N.Y.: Harper and Row, 1959), p. 21.

EPILOGUE
NOTES

1. The general strategy here is inspired by John Rawls' "veil of ignorance," in his **A Theory of Justice,** (Chapter 13, note 14).

2. F.H. Bradley, **Ethical Studies,** (London: Oxford University Press, 1962), p. 190.

3. I am following the logic of Willam James' famous "Will to Believe," (Chapter 1, note 12).

SELECTED BIBLIOGRAPHY

Alexander, Leo. "Medical Science Under Dictatorship," **New England Journal of Medicine,** vol. 241, 1949.

Annas, George. **The Rights of Hospital Patients.** New York: Avon Books, 1975.

Aquinas, Thomas. **Summa Theologica.** New York: Benziger, 1947.

Aristotle. **Nichomachean Ethics;** (ed. by Martin Ostwald). Indianapolis: The Liberal Arts Press, 1962.

Augustine. **Confessions;** (trans. by R.S. Pine-Coffin). New York: Penguin Books, 1961.

Ayer, A.J. **Language Truth and Logic.** New York: Dover, 1952.

Bandman, E. and Bandman B. (eds.) **Bioethics and Human Rights.** Boston: Little Brown, 1978.

Blank, R.H. **The Political Implications of Human Genetic Technology.** Colorado: Westview Press, 1981.

Becker, Ernest. **The Denial of Death.** New York: Macmillan, 1973.

Beecher, Henry K. "Ethics and Clinical Research," **New England Journal of Medicine,** vol. 274, 1966.

Bok, Sissela. **Lying.** New York: Vintage Books, 1979.

Bontempo, Charles and S. Jack Odell. **The Owl of Minerva.** New York: McGraw-Hill, 1975.

Bradley, F.H. **Ethical Studies.** London: Oxford University Press, 1962.

Broad, C.D. **Ethics and the History of Philosophy.** London: Routledge and Kegan Paul, 1952.

Brownlie, Ian. (ed.) **Basic Documents on Human Rights.** Oxford: Clarendon Press, 1981.

Bruening, W.M. **The Is-Ought Problem: its History, Analysis and Dissolution.** Washington: University Press of America, 1978.

Callahan, Daniel. "The WHO Definition of Health," **Hastings Center Studies,** vol. 1, no. 3, 1973.

Campbell, C.A. **In Defence of Free Will.** London: Allen and Unwin, 1967.

Camus, Albert. **The Myth of Sisyphus and Other Essays.** New York: Alfred A. Knopf, 1955.

Capron, Alexander. "A Functional Approach to Informed Consent," **University of Pennsylvania Law Review,** vol. 123, 1974.

Cohen, Howard. **Equal Rights for Children.** New Jersey: Rowman and Littlefield, 1980.

Dewey, John. **Democracy and Education.** New York: Free Press, 1966.

_____. **The Moral Writings of John Dewey;** (ed. by James Gouinlock). New York: Hafner Press, 1976.

_____. **Reconstruction in Philosophy.** Boston: Beacon Press, 1957.

Dougherty, Charles J. and Sandra L. Dougherty. "Moral Reconstruction in the Hospital: A Legal and Philosophical Perspective on Patient Rights," **Creighton Law Review,** vol. 14, no. 4 (supp.), 1981.

Dougherty, Charles J. "The Right to Health Care: First Aid in the Emergency Room," Public Law Forum, vol. 4, no. 1, 1984.

Draper, Thomas. (ed.) **Human Rights.** New York: H.W. Wilson, 1982.

Dworkin, Ronald. **Taking Rights Seriously.** Cambridge: Harvard University Press, 1977.

Edwards, Paul. (ed.) **Encyclopedia of Philosophy.** New York: Macmillan and the Free Press, 1967.

Engelhardt, H. Tristram, Jr. and Daniel Callahan. (eds.) **Science, Ethics and Medicine.** New York: Hastings Center, 1976.

Fingarette, Herbert. **Self-deception.** New York: Humanities Press, 1969.

Frankena, William. **Ethics.** New Jersey: Prentice-Hall, 1973.

Freund, Paul. (ed.) **Experimentation With Human Subjects.** New York: George Braziller, 1964.

Fried, Charles. **Right and Wrong.** Cambridge: Harvard University Press, 1978.

Goldman, Alan. **The Moral Foundations of Professional Ethics.** New Jersey: Rowman and Littlefield, 1980.

Hare, R.M. **The Language of Morals.** Oxford: Oxford University Press, 1964.

_____. **Freedom and Reason.** Oxford: Clarendon Press, 1963.

Hart, H.L.A. "Are There Any Natural Rights?" **Philosophical Review,** vol. 64, 1955.

Heidegger, Martin. **Being and Time;** (trans. by J. Marquarrie and E. Robinson). New York: Harper and Row, 1962.

Hempel, Carl. **The Philosophy of Natural Science.** New Jersey: Prentice-Hall, 1966.

Henkin, Louis. **The Rights of Man Today.** Colorado: Westview Press, 1978.

Hilton, Bruce, et al. (eds.) **Ethical Issues in Human Genetics: Genetic Counseling and the Use of Genetic Knowledge.** New York: Phenum Publishing, 1973.

Hook, Sidney. **Philosophy and Public Policy.** Carbondale: Southern Illinois University Press, 1980.

Hudson, W.D. (ed.) **The Is-Ought Problem.** London: Macmillan, 1969.

Husserl, Edmund. **Logical Investigations;** (trans. by J.N. Findlay). New York: Humanities Press, 1970.

Illich, Ivan. **Medical Nemesis.** New York: Pantheon, 1976.

James, William. **Pragmatism and Four Essays from the Meaning of Truth;** (ed. by Ralph Barton Perry). New York: Meridan Press, 1955.

Jonsen, A.R. "History of Medical Ethics," **Encyclopedia of Bioethics;** (ed. by Warren T. Reich). New York: Free Press, 1978.

Kant, Immanuel. **Grounding for the Metaphysics of Morals;** (trans. by James W. Ellington). Indianapolis: Hackett, 1981.

Katz, Jay. **Experimentation with Human Beings.** New York: Russell Sage Foundation, 1973.

King, Joseph. **The Law of Medical Malpractice.** St. Paul: West Publishing, 1977.

Kubler-Ross, Elizabeth. **On Death and Dying.** New York: Macmillan, 1969.

Kuhn, Thomas S. **The Structure of Scientific Revolution.** Chicago: University of Chicago Press, 1970.

Lasch, Christopher. **The Culture of Narcissism.** New York: Norton, 1978.

Lauer, Quentin. **Hegel's Concept of God.** Albany: State University of New York Press, 1982.

Levi, Albert William. **Philosophy as Social Expression.** Chicago: University of Chicago Press, 1974.

Lyons, David. **Forms and Limits of Utilitarianism.** Oxford: Clarendon Press, 1965.

Mappes, T. and J. Zembaty. (eds.) **Biomedical Ethics** New York: McGraw-Hill, 1966.

Maritain, Jacques. **The Rights of Man and Natural Law;** (ed. by Doris Anson). New York: Scribner's Sons, 1943.

McCormick, Richard. "To Save or Let Die: The Dilemma of Modern Medicine," **Journal of the American Medical Association,** vol. 229, 1974.

Mead, George Herbert. **Mind, Self and Society.** Chicago: University of Chicago Press, 1962.

Melden, A.I. **Rights and Persons.** Berkeley: University of California Press, 1980.

Mill, John Stuart. **On Liberty.** Indianapolis: Hackett, 1978.

_____. **Utilitarianism;** (ed. by Samuel Gorovitz). Indianapolis: Bobbs-Merrill, 1971.

Moore, G.E. **Principia Ethica.** Cambridge: Cambridge University Press, 1979.

Nagel, Thomas. **Mortal Questions.** Cambridge: Cambridge University Press, 1979.

Nesbit, Robert. **History of the Idea of Progress.** New York: Basic Books, 1980.

Outka, Gene. "Social Justice and Equal Access to Health Care," **Journal of Religious Ethics,** vol. 2, no. 1, 1974.

Parsons, Talcott. **The Social System.** New York: Free Press, 1951.

Passmore, John. **The Perfectibility of Man.** New York: Scribner Sons, 1971.

Peirce, Charles S. **The Collected Papers; Vols. I-VI** (ed. by Charles Hartshorne and Paul Weiss); **Vols. VII-VIII** (ed. by A. Burks). Cambridge: Harvard University Press, 1931 and 1958.

Plato. **The Collected Dialogues;** (ed. by Edith Hamilton and Huntington Cairns). Princeton: Princeton University Press, 1969.

Potter, Vincent. **Charles S. Peirce on Norms and Ideals.** Boston: Massachusetts University Press, 1967.

Powledge, Tabitha. "Genetic Screening," **Encyclopedia of Bioethics** (ed. by Warren T. Reich) New York: Free Press, 1978.

Pritchard, H.A. "Does Moral Philosophy Rest on a Mistake?" in **Readings in Ethical Theory;** (ed. by Wilfred Sellars and John Hospers). New Jersey: Prentice-Hall, 1970.

Ramsey, Paul. **Patient as Person.** New Haven: Yale University Press, 1970.

Rawls, John. **A Theory of Justice.** Cambridge: Harvard University Press, 1971.

Rosenbaum, Alan, M. **The Philosophy of Human Rights.** Connecticut: Greenwood Press, 1980.

Royce, Josiah. **The World and the Individual.** New York: Macmillan, 1901.

Ryle, Gilbert. **The Concept of Mind.** New York: Barnes and Noble, 1949.

Sartre, John Paul. **Existentialism and Human Emotions.** New York: Philosophical Library, 1957.

Sen, Amartya. **Utilitarianism and Beyond.** Cambridge: Cambridge University Press, 1982.

Shue, Henry. **Basic Rights.** Princeton: Princeton University Press, 1980.

Singer, Peter. **Practical Ethics.** Cambridge: Cambridge University Press, 1979.

Smart, J.J.C. and B. Williams. (eds.) **Utilitarianism, For and Against.** Cambridge: Cambridge University Press, 1973.

Starr, Paul. **The Social Transformation of American Medicine.** New York: Basic Books, 1982.

Stevenson, Charles. "The Emotive Meaning of Ethical Terms," **Mind,** Vol. 46, 1937.

Vaihinger, Hans. **The Philosophy of As If;** (trans. by C.K. Ogden). New York: Harcourt Brace, 1952.

Vardin, Patricia and Ilene Brady. (eds.) **Children's Rights.** New York: Teachers College Press, 1979.

Warnock, Mary. **Existentialism.** London: Oxford University Press, 1970.

Werner, E.E. **Cross-Cultural Child Development.** California: Brooks/ Cole, 1979.

Whitehead, Alfred North. **Nature and Life.** Chicago: University Press, 1938.

Winner, Langdon. **Autonomous Technology.** Cambridge: MIT Press, 1977.

Wittgenstein, Ludwig. **Philosophical Investigations;** (trans. by G. Anscombe). New York: Macmillan, 1968.